PULMONARY AND RESPIRATORY DISEASES AND DISORDERS

CYSTIC AND IDIOPATHIC PULMONARY FIBROSIS

RISK FACTORS, MANAGEMENT AND LONG-TERM HEALTH OUTCOMES

Pulmonary and Respiratory Diseases and Disorders

Additional books in this series can be found on Nova's website under the Series tab.

Additional e-books in this series can be found on Nova's website under the e-book tab.

PULMONARY AND RESPIRATORY DISEASES AND DISORDERS

CYSTIC AND IDIOPATHIC PULMONARY FIBROSIS

RISK FACTORS, MANAGEMENT AND LONG-TERM HEALTH OUTCOMES

LORENZO ROBERTSON
EDITOR

New York

Library of Congress Cataloging-in-Publication Data

ISBN: 978-1-63485-508-2
Library of Congress Control Number: 2016942393

Published by Nova Science Publishers, Inc. † New York

CONTENTS

PREFACE

Cystic fibrosis (CF) is one of the most common autosomal recessive disorders in the Caucasian population with an estimated incidence of 1 in 2,500 childbirths. While this disease affects several organ systems of the body, morbidity and mortality is chiefly related to the extent of pulmonary involvement. Idiopathic pulmonary fibrosis (IPF) is the most common idiopathic interstitial disease of the lung of unknown etiology with a median survival time of about 3 years. IPF occurs mainly in men older than 60 years who have comorbidities such as pulmonary hypertension, COPD, lung cancer, gastro-esophageal reflux, ischemic heart disease and obstructive sleep apnoea. This book provides current research on risk factors of CF and IPF, as well as management options and long-term health outcomes of the disorders.

Chapter 1 - This multisystem inherited disorder is a consequence of genetic mutations which result in defective functioning of the cystic fibrosis transmembrane conductance regulator (*CFTR*) chloride channel. Being a complex glycoprotein (1,480 amino acids) encoded by approximately 250,000 base pairs, more than 2,000 different mutations have been described in the gene encoding for this protein in patients with CF. Manifestations of CF include bronchiectasis, sinonasal polyposis, chronic pancreatitis with pancreatic insufficiency (fat malabsorption, fat-soluble vitamin deficiencies and diabetes mellitus), intestinal pathology (meconium ileus, intestinal atresia), osteoporosis, malnutrition, failure to thrive, infertility and delayed puberty, all of which culminate in an overall reduced life expectancy. While this disease affects several organ systems of the body, morbidity and mortality is chiefly related to the extent of pulmonary involvement. Management of patients with this disorder is best carried out by dedicated teams in specialized centers and involves education of patients and their families, close monitoring and regular follow-up, salt supplementation, treatment of pulmonary infections and exacerbations (antibiotics, pulmonary toilet, ventilatory support, bronchodilators and mucolytics), pancreatic enzyme replacement and nutritional support, screening for diabetes mellitus, assessment of bone health, endocrine evaluation and hormone replacement, assisted reproductive technologies, and rehabilitative support. Novel treatment strategies for CF employ small molecules for correcting *CFTR* defects at the molecular level by enhancing protein folding and expression (*CFTR* correctors), or potentiating *CFTR* channel activation (*CFTR* potentiators). More recently, a combination of *CFTR* corrector and potentiator molecules (viz. lumacaftor–ivacaftor) was approved by the Food and Drug Administration for CF patients homozygous for the ΔF508 mutation. While such treatment options can potentially revolutionize the treatment of CF, their cost-benefit balance is yet to be established. Several outcome measures and clinical assessment tools have been reported in the literature for monitoring patients with CF and predicting their prognosis. Current best evidence suggests that prognosis for individual patients may be affected by gender, type of genetic mutation, body mass index, pulmonary function (as assessed by forced expiratory volume in 1 second—FEV_1), nasal potential difference (NPD) or sweat chloride concentration at diagnosis, CF-related diabetes mellitus, CF-related liver disease, and airway microbiome composition. Newborn and prenatal carrier screening programs are currently being offered in many parts of the globe and have been effective in decreasing the incidence of CF substantially. Overall life expectancy for patients with CF has improved over the past decade with a median expected survival of 37 years. With the development of targeted genetic therapies, prognosis for patients with CF will continue to improve even further.

Chapter 2 - Liver disease (LD) in cystic fibrosis (CF) has become a matter of greater concern since the population of CF patients lives longer. Early recognition of LD in CF is not easy because its onset is often insidious and clinical, biochemical, and other indicators are relatively insensitive.

Aims: The study analyses the prevalence of CF-related LD in Macedonian CF population and the clinical and genetic characteristics of these patients, in an attempt to find out the possible risk factors for its development.

Methods: All patients older than 2 years (n= 102) were screened for LD through clinical, biochemical, ehographic, and hepatobiliary scintigraphic assessment. LD was defined by the finding of hepatomegaly and/or splenomegaly; significant and persistent increase of at least two serum liver enzyme levels, suggestive ultrasonographic abnormalities (score >4), and morphologic or functional scintigraphic abnormalities.

Results: According to predefined criteria, 33 patients (32.3%) were classified as having LD, three of them with portal hypertension. The clinical presentations of LD had 13, abnormal liver blood test results 21, ultrasound abnormalities 33, and scintigraphic abnormalities 22 of the patients. A male predominance was found in the group with LD (69.7%). Pancreatic insufficiency was present in all patients with LD. There was no significant difference in the pulmonary function, nutritional status, and in the prevalence of meconium ileus or DIOS between groups with and without LD. Genetic analysis showed higher frequency of F508del mutation in LD group (77.3%) vs. no LD group (66.2%). All patients with LD had ″severe″ mutations: F508del, G542X, N1303K, 621+G→T, R1066C, CFTRdel.21Kb, 1811+1G→C, V456F, R1162X, 457TAT→G, and Y161D.

Conclusion: Male CF patients who have pancreatic insufficiency and carry mutations associated with a severe phenotype are in increased risk to develop LD. Regular screening for LD and identification of patients with liver involvement is of great important in management of CF patients. The authors' data highlight the value of ultrasound as the most sensitive tool for detection and follow up patents with LD.

Chapter 3 - Although the benefits of lung transplantation for young children with cystic fibrosis (CF) remains somewhat controversial, lung transplantation is the only therapeutic option that is likely to improve survival and quality of life for children and adult patients with CF who have advanced bronchiectatic lung disease and progressive respiratory failure that is unresponsive to other therapies. If patients wish to be candidates for lung transplantation, the appearance of signs of impending respiratory failure should trigger referral to a transplant center where a lung transplant team can determine whether criteria for lung transplantation are met and whether potential recipients lack absolute contraindications for transplantation. Major obstacles to long-term survival of lung transplant recipients include peri-operative complications, infections, and the development of chronic lung allograft dysfunction (CLAD). However, despite the many potential complications of lung transplantation, recipients can have prolonged survival and good quality of life. This chapter reviews referral criteria, contraindications to lung transplantation, and candidate evaluation and listing. Additionally, technical aspects of donor lung implantation, principles of peri-operative and post-transplant management, and long-term outcomes are discussed.

Chapter 4 - Cystic fibrosis (CF) is a lethal monogenic disease with an early mortality and morbidity. It is caused by mutations in the gene encoding the cystic fibrosis transmembrane conductance regulator (CFTR) that engenders thick, sticky mucus to form in the lungs, pancreas, and other organs. Survival and quality of life have improved, through better management of nutrition and, respiratory infections, rather than through interventions that target the basic defect. In fact, therapy for CF has progressed during the past several decades. Withal, with more than 2000 mutations that can produce a faulty CFTR, the management of CF remains a challenge. Several innovative drugs recently approved by the Food and Drug Administration, termed genetic modulators, target the underlying disease by modulating the CFTR defect.

Nowadays, many innovations have concerned the daily treatment of CF, focus on inhaled and oral medications and optimized nutrition, such as the development of drugs with "intelligent nebulisers" and dry-powder inhalers becoming commonplace. These developments have occurred in conjunction with development of a wider variety of therapeutic strategies. In fact, new therapeutic strategies have been developed to target various aspects of the physiological waterfall in CF. The development of Oral agents such as ivacaftor, which work for selected genotypes to directly potentiate the cystic fibrosis transmembrane conductance regulator (CFTR) protein and lumacaftor to correct intracellular processing of CFTR offer huge potential to target the underlying defects in specific CFTR mutations and alter the disease process, and could be life-changing. The vast majority of efforts over the last 20 years have focused on developing a gene therapy for CF lung disease largely due to the urgent need for more effective treatments and the noninvasive accessibility of the lung also the gene therapy approach is potential use in all mutation classes.

Over the past few decades, remarkable improvements have been made in clinical outcomes for CF patients including better nutritional status, new target and gene therapy. Many drug have also been developed to improve the quality of life of patients.

Chapter 5 - Background: Murine models can be useful for understanding complex diseases such as pulmonary fibrosis. Bleomycin, administered via a wide variety of routes, is commonly used to induce lung fibrosis in rodents. The authors compared fibrotic responses in the lung elicited by bleomycin given by subcutaneous injection and intratracheal administration. Mice were treated with one dose of intratracheal bleomycin or with subcutaneous bleomycin daily for 14 days. Lungs and skin were analyzed for fibrosis by histopathology and immunostaining for alpha-smooth muscle actin, and transforming growth factor-beta protein level and apoptosis were evaluated. Results: While intratracheal and subcutaneous approaches yielded comparable severity of pulmonary fibrosis, distinct spatial and temporal evolution of pulmonary changes was noted. Intratracheal bleomycin induced early onset and rapid resolution of inflammation, while subcutaneous bleomycin caused more sustained lung inflammation with slow resolution of injury. Moreover, subcutaneous bleomcyin caused a predominantly peri-vascular pattern of lung fibrosis, whereas intratracheal instillation of bleomycin additionally caused injury around the airways. Early apoptotic responses were primarily centered around the airways in mice given intratracheal bleomycin but were seen around blood vessels with subcutaneous bleomycin. Conclusions: Subcutaneous administration of bleomycin causes a pattern of lung injury and fibrosis that is histologically distinct from that induced by the intratracheal route. These two distinct modes of bleomycin delivery might have utility for modeling interstitial lung disease associated with airway injury, such as idiopathic pulmonary fibrosis, versus systemic autoimmunity, such as systemic sclerosis.

Chapter 6 - Idiopathic pulmonary fibrosis (IPF) is the most common idiopathic interstitial disease of the lung of unknown etiology with a median survival time of about 3 years. IPF occurs mainly in men older than 60 years who have comorbidities such as pulmonary hypertension, COPD, lung cancer, gastro-esophageal reflux, ischemic heart disease and obstructive sleep apnoea. IPF affects the quality of life (QL) by fatigue mostly associated with poor sleep quality. In IPF patients alteration in sleep architecture, increased sleep fragmentation and slow wave sleep periods are detectable. During the vulnerable REM sleep stage sleep related hypoventilation and obstructive sleep apnea syndrome are often observed. These sleep disorders in IPF are associated with reduction of QL and increased risk of mortality. Therefore, clinicians should refer patients with IPF to sleep centers for the diagnosis and possible treatment of sleep related disorders with continuous positive airway pressure devices. In the absence of an effective therapy for IPF, the treatment of sleep disorders could significantly improve the QL of these patients.

Chapter 7 - Idiopathic pulmonary fibrosis (IPF) is a progressive lung disease determined by dysfunction of epithelial cells. Basically normal parenchyma is subverted into fibrotic tissue useless for gas exchange.

Genetic factors, aging and the exposure to exogenous agents are involved in the beginning of the disorder process. The genetic determination gained importance when plenty of evidences have been highlighted like familial clustering, combination with rare genetic disorders, and variability of IPF onset on individuals with same agents exposures where highlighted. MUC5 B variants are associated with the disorder, while TOLLIP and SPPL2C variants are related to IPF susceptibility and mortality. At the moment, the determination of genetic variants cannot be a routine exam and, at the same time would not be useful in therapy or in prognosis since its role is limited to IPF predisposition.

Predisposition is only the first of the three IPF pathogenesis stages.

The second stage sees the onset of profibrotic processes: the consequences of excessive TGF β activation, Endoplasmic Reticulum stress and growth factors secretion are the epithelial to mesenchymal transition (EMT) and fibrocyte recruitment. The last stage is the progression with pathologic fibroblast differentiation and matrix remodeling ending in epigenetic changes that can feed itself the disease development activating persistently mesenchymal cells and simulating fibrosis progression.

The differentiation stage is useful to determine molecular pathways and address IPF therapies towards specific targets.

Latest studies demonstrated the relationship between N-acetylcysteine (NAC) and EMT, MUC5 ac, MUC5B and TOLLIP. The use of acetylcysteine seems to be favourable in patient's therapy, at least in some genetic cluster. In the light of these latest findings NAC should be reconsidered in IPF therapy.

In: Cystic and Idiopathic Pulmonary Fibrosis ISBN: 978-1-63485-508-2
Editor: Lorenzo Robertson

Chapter 1

CLINICAL MANIFESTATIONS OF CYSTIC FIBROSIS AND THEIR MANAGEMENT

Ibrahim A. Janahi*[1,*], *MD, FCCP, FRCPCH and Abdul Rehman*[2], *MD

[1] Professor of Clinical Pediatrics, Weill-Cornell Medical College–Qatar; Division Chief, Pediatric Pulmonology, Department of Pediatrics, Hamad Medical Corporation, Doha, Qatar

[2] Resident Physician, Internal Medicine Section, Department of Medicine, Hamad Medical Corporation, Doha, Qatar

ABSTRACT

Cystic fibrosis (CF) is one of the most common autosomal recessive disorders in the Caucasian population with an estimated incidence of 1 in 2,500 childbirths. This multisystem inherited disorder is a consequence of genetic mutations which result in defective functioning of the cystic fibrosis transmembrane conductance regulator (*CFTR*) chloride channel. Being a complex glycoprotein (1,480 amino acids) encoded by approximately 250,000 base pairs, more than 2,000 different mutations have been described in the gene encoding for this protein in patients with CF. Manifestations of CF include bronchiectasis, sinonasal polyposis, chronic pancreatitis with pancreatic insufficiency (fat malabsorption, fat-

---

* Corresponding Author: Prof. Dr. Ibrahim A. Janahi, Senior Consultant and Division Chief, Pediatric Pulmonology, Hamad Medical Corporation, P.O. box 3050, Doha, Qatar. Tel: (+974) 4439 2551. Fax: (+974) 4439 571. Email: ijanahi@hamad.qa.

soluble vitamin deficiencies and diabetes mellitus), intestinal pathology (meconium ileus, intestinal atresia), osteoporosis, malnutrition, failure to thrive, infertility and delayed puberty, all of which culminate in an overall reduced life expectancy. While this disease affects several organ systems of the body, morbidity and mortality is chiefly related to the extent of pulmonary involvement. Management of patients with this disorder is best carried out by dedicated teams in specialized centers and involves education of patients and their families, close monitoring and regular follow-up, salt supplementation, treatment of pulmonary infections and exacerbations (antibiotics, pulmonary toilet, ventilatory support, bronchodilators and mucolytics), pancreatic enzyme replacement and nutritional support, screening for diabetes mellitus, assessment of bone health, endocrine evaluation and hormone replacement, assisted reproductive technologies, and rehabilitative support. Novel treatment strategies for CF employ small molecules for correcting *CFTR* defects at the molecular level by enhancing protein folding and expression (*CFTR* correctors), or potentiating *CFTR* channel activation (*CFTR* potentiators). More recently, a combination of *CFTR* corrector and potentiator molecules (viz. lumacaftor–ivacaftor) was approved by the Food and Drug Administration for CF patients homozygous for the ΔF508 mutation. While such treatment options can potentially revolutionize the treatment of CF, their cost-benefit balance is yet to be established. Several outcome measures and clinical assessment tools have been reported in the literature for monitoring patients with CF and predicting their prognosis. Current best evidence suggests that prognosis for individual patients may be affected by gender, type of genetic mutation, body mass index, pulmonary function (as assessed by forced expiratory volume in 1 second—FEV_1), nasal potential difference (NPD) or sweat chloride concentration at diagnosis, CF-related diabetes mellitus, CF-related liver disease, and airway microbiome composition. Newborn and prenatal carrier screening programs are currently being offered in many parts of the globe and have been effective in decreasing the incidence of CF substantially. Overall life expectancy for patients with CF has improved over the past decade with a median expected survival of 37 years. With the development of targeted genetic therapies, prognosis for patients with CF will continue to improve even further.

Keywords: cystic fibrosis, *CFTR* gene, management, pathophysiology

List of Abbreviations

^{18}FDG	^{18}Fluorodeoxyglucose
AAV	Adeno-associated virus

ABC	ATP-binding cassette
AP-1	Activator protein-1
ASL	Airway surface liquid
BMD	Bone mineral density
cAMP	3′,5′-cyclic adenosine monophosphate
CAVD	Congenital absence of the vas deferens
CBP/p300	cAMP response element-binding protein
C/EBP	CCAAT-enhancer binding protein
CF	Cystic fibrosis
CFRD	Cystic fibrosis related diabetes
CFTR	Cystic fibrosis transmembrane conductance regulator
CFF-TDN	Cystic Fibrosis Foundation-Therapeutics Development Network
CIP	CFTR-interacting protein
CRP	C-reactive protein
CT	Computed tomography
DIOS	Distal intestinal obstruction syndrome
DNA	Deoxyribonucleic acid
ENaC	Epithelial sodium channel
ER	Endoplasmic reticulum
ERAD	ER-associated degradation
$FEF_{25–75\%}$	Forced expiratory flow at 25–75% of forced vital capacity
$FEF_{75\%}$	Forced expiratory flow when 75% of forced vital capacity has been exhaled
FEV_1	Forced expiratory volume in 1 second
FRC	Functional residual capacity
FVC	Functional vital capacity
HDAC	Histone deacetylase
HNF1	Hepatocyte nuclear factor 1
ICM	Intestinal current measurement
LCI	Lung clearance index
MBW	Multiple breath washout
miRNA	Micro-ribonucleic acid
MRI	Magnetic resonance imaging
mRNA	Messenger ribonucleic acid
MRSA	Methicillin-resistant *Staphylococcus aureus*
NBD	Nucleotide binding domain
NIPPV	Non-invasive positive pressure ventilation
NPD	Nasal potential difference

OGTT	Oral glucose tolerance test
P/CAF	CBP-associated factor
PET	Positron emission tomography
PKA	Protein kinase A
RVRTC	Raised volume rapid thoracoabdominal compression
siRNA	Small interfering ribonucleic acid
TMD	Transmembrane domain
UTR	Untranslated region

INTRODUCTION

Cystic fibrosis (CF) is an inherited multisystem disorder caused by genetic mutations in the cystic fibrosis transmembrane conductance regulator (*CFTR*) gene [1]. *CFTR* protein is a chloride channel expressed in various tissues of the body including epithelia of respiratory and gastrointestinal tracts, pancreas, vas deferens and sweat glands [2]. Being involved in transport of sodium, chloride and bicarbonate ions, defective functioning of *CFTR* results in pleiotropic effects on several organ systems of the body and accounts for substantial morbidity and mortality for patients with CF. As of now, CF is the most common *life-limiting* autosomal recessive disorder in the Caucasian population [3].

While descriptions of patients with probable CF can be traced back to as early as the eighteenth century, the first formal account of CF as a distinct disorder was reported by Dorothy Andersen in 1938 [4]. The term "cystic fibrosis" was proposed for this disorder based on the typical morphology of the pancreas in such patients, which consists of cysts and areas of fibrosis within the pancreas [5]. The autosomal recessive pattern of this inherited disorder was recognized in 1945 by Hodges and Andersen [6]. Subsequently, the most common mutation for CF (ΔF508) was discovered in 1988, which led to the identification of the gene responsible for CF (i.e., *CFTR*) in 1989 at the Hospital for Sick Children (Toronto) [7, 8].

Over the past few decades, extensive research has been conducted on understanding the pathophysiology and molecular genetics of CF. Hitherto, more than 2,000 different mutations have been described in the *CFTR* gene [9]. While a definitive cure for this disorder still remains elusive, novel drugs and therapies for this genetic disorder are actively being investigated and our understanding of the disease is continuously evolving. Better management of patients with CF has led to a dramatic improvement in overall life expectancy [10]. In the following pages, we describe the molecular biology, pathophysiology, management and prognosis of patients with CF in the light of currently available evidence.

EPIDEMIOLOGY

The incidence of CF in different ethnic groups varies considerably and the epidemiology of this disease has been changing over time due to a number of factors. CF is the most common lethal genetic disorder in the European population with an estimated incidence of 1 in 2,000–3,000 live births [11]. The highest incidence of CF has been recorded at 1 in 1,353 live births in Ireland. In the United States, the incidence of CF has been shown to be about 1 in 3,300–3,500 live births [12]. In contrast, the incidence of CF in Asian and African children is considerably lower. Among African American and Asian American children, only 1 in 15,000 and 1 in 31,000 suffer from CF respectively [13].

Being an autosomal recessive disorder, inheritance of two mutated alleles is required to express the disease phenotype. Heterozygous carriers of the mutated *CFTR* allele are typically asymptomatic and may be detected only through genetic screening. The frequency of the CF allele is as common as 1 in 25 in people of European descent and 1 in 30 in American Caucasians [14]. Despite being a lethal mutation, carriage of the ΔF508 mutation in the Caucasian population is astounding. Heterozygote advantage of ΔF508 carriers against cholera and typhoid fever has been hypothesized [15]. However, there is little evidence to corroborate this claim.

CF is diagnosed with nearly equal frequency in both men and women. However, women generally tend to have a worse survival when compared with men [16]. Some studies suggested that hormonal differences (estrogen) may play a role, although the exact mechanism remains unclear [17]. Likewise, data from the European Cystic Fibrosis Society shows that household income has a significant association with mortality rates. A household income of less than $20,000 per year is associated with a 44% increase in mortality in CF patients when compared with those with a household income of more than $50,000 per year [18]. This disparity in survival persists even after accounting for differences in access to treatment facilities and may be related to diverse factors, such as over-crowding and environmental pollution [19].

The incidence and prevalence of CF in the population has changed over time owing to increased survival of patients, earlier age at diagnosis and improved programmes of carrier and newborn screening [20]. Worldwide, close to 100,000 individuals are affected by CF, while, in the United States, the prevalence of CF is estimated at 1 in 10,000 [21]. The median predicted survival for patients with CF has been constantly improving and is currently estimated to be 37 years. Data from the Cystic Fibrosis Foundation registry shows that patients diagnosed by screening have a better overall survival as compared to those diagnosed by symptoms [22]. In a large population-based study in Italy, Castellani and colleagues showed that carrier screening was associated with a decrease in the incidence of CF by 4–24% [23].

Molecular Biology

CFTR Gene

The *CFTR* gene was first identified on the long arm of chromosome 7 (7q31) by positional cloning techniques in 1989 [24]. This gene is composed of 27 exons and spans almost 190 kb of genomic deoxyribonucleic acid (DNA). Belonging to the traffic ATPase family of genes, transcription of this important gene is tightly regulated both spatially and temporally [25]. The promoter sequence of this gene is special in that it possesses multiple transcriptional start sites, but lacks a TATA box sequence. The promoter sequence also contains 3′,5′-cyclic adenosine monophosphate (cAMP) response elements, glucocorticoid response elements, a CCAAT-enhancer binding protein (C/EBP) binding site, and Sp1 and activator protein-1 (AP-1) binding sites [26]. These promoter sequences are important in maintaining normal *CFTR* gene transcription and a T to G substitution in the AP-1 binding site (located at position –741 from the *CFTR* gene cap site) can be detected in certain mutant *CFTR* genes [27]. The degree of promoter region CpG methylation also affects *CFTR* expression with high levels of CpG methylation typically seen in tissues with low level of *CFTR* gene transcription [28]. In addition to the promoter sequence, at least 9 other regions (introns 1, 2, 3, 10, 16, 17a, 18, 20 and 21) are also involved in regulating transcription of this gene [29]. Apart from these sequences, several transcription factors can affect transcription of the *CFTR* gene including hepatocyte nuclear factor 1 (HNF1), cAMP response element–binding protein (CBP/p300) and CBP–associated factor (P/CAF) [30]. The importance of understanding the regulation of *CFTR* gene expression is that only a small increase in *CFTR* gene expression in affected individuals can ameliorate symptoms of CF [31].

CFTR Biosynthesis

Transcription of the *CFTR* gene results in the formation of a messenger ribonucleic acid (mRNA) that is 6.5 kb long and contains a 1.5 kb 3′ UTR (untranslated region). Transcription of the *CFTR* gene itself can regulate the amount of *CFTR* mRNA transcripts in the cell [32]. Moreover, alternative splicing of the *CFTR* mRNA transcripts is another cellular mechanism by which *CFTR* function is modulated. More recently, different types of micro-ribonucleic acids (miRNA) have been shown to interact with the 3′ UTR region of *CFTR* mRNA transcripts and affect their translation; the most notable of these miRNAs are hsa-miR-145 and hsa-miR-494 [33].

Following export from the nucleus, the *CFTR* mRNA transcript is translated on polyribosomes and the nascent polypeptide chain undergoes significant co-translational and post-translational modifications prior to reaching the apical membrane surface of epithelial cells [34]. As soon as the *CFTR* nascent polypeptide emerges from ribosomes, it is folded in a highly coordinated manner in three distinct cellular compartments (i.e., endoplasmic reticulum [ER] membrane, ER lumen, and cytosol). This process of protein folding is coordinated by complex "quality control" cellular machinery that includes chaperones (Hsp70, Hsp40, and Hsp90), calnexin, BAP31, Csps, CHIP and other proteins [35]. Based on experimental studies, *CFTR* biosynthesis has been estimated to take 9–10 minutes, while complete folding of the polypeptide into its final protein form has been estimated to take 30–120 minutes [36]. If the *CFTR* polypeptide fails to achieve its normal conformational configuration, chaperones (such as Hsp70) recruit E3 and E4 ubiquitin ligases that ubiquitinate the newly formed polypeptide and tag it for degradation by the 26S proteasome [37]. Experimental studies have shown that as much as 75% of the wild type *CFTR* polypeptide undergoes ubiquitination and subsequent degradation due to improper folding [38]. In patients carrying the ΔF508 mutation (the most common mutation implicated in CF), nearly 99% of the *CFTR* polypeptide undergoes degradation due to ER-associated degradation (ERAD) [39].

Apart from protein folding, the *CFTR* polypeptide undergoes core glycosylation, oligomerization and maturation within the ER lumen. Following exit from the ER, the *CFTR* protein is fully glycosylated within the Golgi complex and traverses a number of complex pathways prior to its insertion within the apical cell membrane surface [40]. A number of *CFTR* interacting proteins (CIP) have been identified that affect *CFTR* trafficking within the cell and its transport to the apical cell membrane surface in epithelial cells.

Of these, the most prominent ones are SNAREs, Rabs and EBP50 [41]. Understanding the role of these CIPs is crucial to understanding the diverse physiologic functions of the *CFTR* protein and its phenotypic manifestations in patients with different types of *CFTR* mutations [42].

Structure of CFTR

CFTR is a polytopic glycoprotein belonging to the ABCC7 transporter family and is composed of 1480 amino acid. This membrane protein has an elaborate structure that is formed by five distinct domains [43]. Two six-spanning transmembrane domains (TMD1 and TMD2) form the ion channel pore, while another two cytosolic domains (NBD1 and NBD2) are responsible for channel gating and protein folding within the ER. The fifth domain (viz. regulatory [R] domain) is intrinsically unstructured and controls activity of the ion channel through (protein kinase A [PKA]-mediated) phosphorylation [44]. The most common CF mutation (ΔF508) results in the removal of a phenylalanine residue from the NBD1 domain, which reduces folding efficiency of the nascent CFTR polypeptide and results in its ERAD. Moreover, this also reduces the interaction between NBD1 and TMD2 domains, which disrupts normal protein structure and adversely affects channel gating [45].

Overview of CFTR Function

CFTR is a member of the ABC (ATP-binding cassette) family of transporter proteins and is primarily responsible for the transepithelial transport of chloride ions. Sodium ions and water molecules generally follow the flow of chloride ions. Depending on the type of tissue and direction of flow of ions, secretion or reabsorption of sodium chloride and water occurs through the CFTR channel. As an example, reabsorption of salt in sweat glands allows the formation of hypotonic sweat for secretion onto the skin [46]. Likewise, secretion of salt and water from the airway mucus cells is responsible for maintaining normal hydration of the airway surface liquid (ASL) and preventing the formation of viscid mucus gels [47].

Additionally, CFTR channel also plays an important role in controlling bicarbonate secretion as it is permeable to bicarbonate ions itself and indirectly stimulates Cl^-/HCO_3^- exchangers. This function is particularly important in pancreatic tissue as bicarbonate is a major driver of pancreatic duct fluid secretion [48]. Likewise, in gastrointestinal tract, bicarbonate secretion from Brunner's glands is responsible for neutralization of gastric acid [49]. Moreover, even in airway and other epithelial tissues, secretion of bicarbonate ions influences local pH and affects the function of certain proteins (such as prostatin and SPLUNC1) that modulate the secretion of sodium ions from epithelial sodium channels (ENaC). Additionally, bicarbonate ions contribute to innate immunity by maintaining a neutral pH in local tissues [50].

CFTR also plays an integral role in maintaining the normal composition of mucus layer. Mucus, a viscous colloid composed of mucin glycoproteins and antibacterial substances, plays a key role in mucosal immunity [51]. Within goblet cells and submucosal glands, mucins are packaged in secretory vesicles and form a complex with calcium ions. Once mucins are secreted onto the epithelial surface, neutral pH of the local tissues allow bicarbonate ions to complex with calcium ions and unmask negative charges on the mucin molecules. Repulsion by negative charges within mucin molecules accounts for slipperiness and creates a lubricating effect [52]. In patients with CF, defective functioning of CFTR protein results in abnormal bicarbonate secretion and alters the local pH, which results in viscid mucus secretions and defective functioning of mucociliary apparatus [53].

CFTR also protects epithelial surfaces against dysbiosis (i.e., alteration of microbiome) indirectly through control of bicarbonate ion secretion [54]. As mentioned before, neutral pH of local tissues is necessary for the antimicrobial activities of defensins, immunoglobulins and other humoral factors. Experimental studies have shown that a pH-sensitive protein, SPLUNC1, can bind to bacterial lipopolysaccharide and inhibit the growth of *Pseudomonas aeruginosa* [55]. This may explain the observation that patients with CF develop airway colonization with *Pseudomonas aeruginosa*, *Staphylococcus aureus* and other pathogenic organisms [56]. This phenomenon of dysbiosis is not limited to the respiratory epithelium; bacterial overgrowth can also occur within the small intestine. Bacterial overgrowth combined with an ineffective mucus barrier, deranged innate immunity, defective neutralization of gastric acid, impaired formation of micelles and denaturation of pancreatic enzymes all lead to fat malabsorption, reduced intestinal motility and pancreatic insufficiency [57].

PATHOPHYSIOLOGY

The pathophysiology and manifestations of CF are a primary consequence of defective functioning of the *CFTR* chloride channel. This anion channel is expressed in all epithelial tissues of the body and is responsible for the transepithelial transport of chloride, bicarbonate and sodium ions. More recent evidence suggests that *CFTR* may be expressed in non-epithelial tissues of the body (including immune cells, neurons and smooth muscle cells) and this may account for the full spectrum of pathology seen in patients with CF [58]. While the basic structure of the protein is similar in all tissues, its physiologic effects in different tissues of the body are variable and account for diverse clinical manifestations in patients with CF. In the following lines, we review the different types of mutations that may occur in the *CFTR* gene and the consequences of defective functioning of *CFTR* channel in different tissues of the body.

Types of Mutations

As mentioned previously, more than 2,000 mutations in the *CFTR* gene have been described to date [9]. Mutations have been classified into five groups depending on the mechanism by which these mutations affect *CFTR* function [59]. Such mutations may occur either within the coding region (exons) of the *CFTR* gene (most commonly, the nucleotide binding domains [NBD] or R domain), or noncoding regions (such as the promoter sequence). Overall, ΔF508 is the most common mutation and is present in at least one chromosome of 70% of CF patients [7]. Of the remaining mutations, only four (G542X, G551D, N1303K and W1282X) have a frequency of more than 1% [59]. Most of the remaining mutations have been described in individual patients or a single family.

Class I Mutations

Class I mutations affect biosynthesis of *CFTR* and result in the production of a truncated protein or reduced overall biosynthesis. G542X is an example of a class I mutation and results in the creation of a premature termination codon [60]. Most class I mutations result in a severe CF phenotype due to almost negligible levels of *CFTR* functionality. However, some class I mutations (mis-splicing mutations) result in a very mild CF phenotype as they produce a small amount of functional *CFTR* protein that is expressed on epithelial cell membranes [61]. Promoter sequence mutations, which reduce the level of *CFTR* transcription, may also result in a mild CF phenotype as a low level of *CFTR* functionality is retained. Theoretically, patients with class I mutations would be cured through gene replacement therapies. In vivo experiments have suggested that gentamycin treatment may improve *CFTR* function in patients with class I mutations as aminoglycosides can stimulate the suppression of stop codons in various organisms [62].

Class II Mutations

Class II mutations in the *CFTR* gene affect protein maturation by inducing cellular misprocessing of *CFTR* polypeptide. The hallmark of class II mutation is the ΔF508 mutation—the most common mutation in CF patients [7]. As mentioned before, this mutation results in the deletion of a phenylalanine residue from the NBD1 domain, thereby leading to impaired folding of *CFTR* polypeptide and its subsequent degradation within the ER [45]. N1303K mutation is another example of a class II mutation. [63] Theoretically, patients with class II mutations can be rescued by enhancing protein folding or suppressing protein degradation [64].

Class III Mutations

Class III mutations affect *CFTR* channel gating and result in delivery of mutant *CFTR* molecules to the cell membrane, which do not respond to cAMP stimulation. Most such mutations occur within the NBD1 or NBD2 domains of *CFTR*. G551D is an example of a class III mutation [65].

Class IV Mutations

Class IV mutations affect *CFTR* chloride conductance and, similar to class III mutations, result in the delivery of mutant *CFTR* proteins unto the cell membrane. Such *CFTR* proteins undergo normal biosynthesis, cellular trafficking and respond to stimulation by cAMP. However, the magnitude of chloride current generated in response to cAMP stimulation is diminished as compared to normal *CFTR* channels. Class III and IV mutations can be theoretically rectified by increasing the activity of mutant *CFTR* proteins expressed in the plasmalemma of epithelial tissues [68]. R117H [66] and I1234V [67] are examples of class IV mutations. Recently, I1234V mutation has also been suggested to cause a *CFTR* defect similar to class II mutations [67]. These findings indicate the need for further interrogation of *CFTR* mutations to tease out their resultant malfunctions at the molecular and cellular levels in line with precise phenotyping of these mutations.

Class V Mutations

Class V mutations have been now incorporated into class I mutations as they also affect *CFTR* biosynthesis [61]. Typically, class V mutations are mis-splicing mutations and result in the least severe disease phenotype [69]. An example of such mutations is the aberrant splicing of exon 9. Exon 9 normally encodes for the first 21% of NBD1 domain of *CFTR* and is thus crucial for its normal function. However, in patients with aberrant splicing of exon 9, more than 5% of *CFTR* mRNA transcripts containing exon 9 are detectable [70]. This small amount of normal *CFTR* mRNA transcript is sufficient for maintaining normal *CFTR* function and is a proof of the concept that a small increase in *CFTR* function in CF patients can ameliorate the disease phenotype.

Class VI Mutations

Although not accepted by all authorities, Zielenski et al. [71] designated class VI mutations as those mutations that affect *CFTR* protein stability. In normal *CFTR* protein, the C-terminus residues are responsible for maintaining stability of the fully glycosylated *CFTR* protein. In patients with class VI mutations, the *CFTR* molecules undergo normal cellular processing and expression; however, half-life of the mutant protein is reduced manifold. An example of a class VI mutation is Q1412X that results in the removal of 70 residues from the C-terminus of the mutant *CFTR* protein [72].

EFFECT OF CFTR DYSFUNCTION ON VARIOUS TISSUES

Sweat Glands

In normal sweat glands, the mechanism of sweat secretion involves the initial production of a chloride-rich fluid from the acinar cells of the sweat gland, which is modified by the ductal cells to produce a hypotonic fluid for secretion onto the skin [73]. Reabsorption of sodium and chloride (but not water) by the ductal cells is achieved by the *CFTR* channel and is responsible for maintaining the hypotonic composition of normal sweat. The hypotonic composition of normal sweat ensures the delivery of a watery secretion onto the skin for thermoregulation and preserves salt within the vascular compartment under heat stress [74]. In patients with CF, defective functioning of the *CFTR* channel results in impaired reabsorption of chloride from the lumen of the sweat gland duct into the ductal cells. This results in increased excretion of salt in sweat of patients with CF and predisposes them to dehydration and an inability to thermoregulate [75]. This clinical feature of CF was recognized long ago and was recapitulated in the ancient European folkloric saying—*the infant that tastes of salt will surely die* [76]. During the heat wave of 1948 in New York, Di Sant'Agnese recognized the susceptibility of infants with CF to develop heat exhaustion and dehydration. He later discovered that infants with CF had abnormally high levels of sodium and chloride in their sweat [77].

Increased levels of sweat chloride in patients with CF are diagnostically useful and can be detected through pilocarpine-stimulated iontophoresis. A sweat chloride level of more than 60 mEq/L (in patients <20 years of age) or more than 80 mEq/L (in patients $\geq$ 20 years of age) is considered abnormal [78]. An abnormal reading of sweat chloride level should generally be confirmed by a repeat testing. In order to diagnose CF, there should be evidence of chloride channel dysfunction (i.e., abnormal sweat chloride level or nasal potential difference [NPD]) in conjunction with a positive family history of CF, evidence of pancreatic insufficiency, or sino-pulmonary disease consistent with CF [79].

Lung and Small Airways

In patients with CF, *CFTR* dysfunction principally affects the epithelia of the sinuses in the upper airways and bronchial epithelia in the lower airways.

The pathophysiology of abnormal mucus secretion in CF patients has been thoroughly investigated and is believed to be multifactorial and physiologically complex [80]. In simple terms, *CFTR* expressed on the apical surface of epithelial cells is responsible for secretion of chloride ions onto the airway mucosa. Under normal conditions, secretion of chloride is accompanied by transepithelial transport of sodium and water, which leads to hydration of the airway lumen [81]. The mucus layer, being composed of glycoproteins, salts and water, is a complex gel system, in which the viscoelastic properties are primarily accounted for by mucin proteins [47]. Hydration of the mucin glycoproteins is crucial for maintaining normal osmotic pressure of the mucin gel system and ensuring normal transport of mucus along the mucociliary apparatus [81].

In patients with CF, disruption of normal *CFTR* function leads to an inability to secrete chloride ions, which inevitably affects secretion of water and sodium into the airway lumen. Reduced secretion of water into the airway lumen increases the concentration of mucin in the mucus layer and results in a thickened, viscous mucus layer. Such thickened mucus becomes adherent to the ciliary layer of the airway epithelium and results in mucus plugging and blockade of the smaller airways [82]. Moreover, adherent mucus plugs can impair mucociliary clearance, reduce the secretion of anti-microbial proteins (lactoferrin, defensins and lysozymes), activate a pro-inflammatory state in the smaller airways (even in the absence of infection), induce airway remodeling with goblet cell hyperplasia (compounding the problem of mucus plugging), impair oxygenation of airway epithelial cells, lead to an alteration in airway microbiome (dysbiosis) and promote the formation of bacterial biofilms within inspissated mucus [83–86]. Obstruction of the smaller airways by mucus plugs with recurrent pulmonary infections eventually leads to destruction and permanent dilatation of bronchi (bronchiectasis), bronchial stenosis and lung fibrosis. Most patients inevitably develop end-stage lung disease and pulmonary disease accounts for 90% of mortality in CF patients [87, 88].

Paranasal Sinuses

The pathophysiology of thickened mucus secretions in the nasal sinuses is similar to the formation of mucus plugs in the smaller airways. However, in addition to thickened nasal secretions, *CFTR* dysfunction in nasal epithelium leads to other diverse manifestations. *CFTR* anion channel is responsible for secretion of chloride ions into the luminal surface of the nasal mucosa and indirect regulation of sodium transport across the nasal epithelium [89]. Reduced secretion of chloride ions in CF patients leads to the presence of an exaggerated (negative) transepithelial potential difference across the nasal mucosa. This NPD is an indirect measure of the bioelectric properties of the nasal mucosa and can be readily detected by recording the potential difference between an electrode placed beneath the inferior nasal turbinate (on the surface of the nasal mucosa) and an electrode placed in the subcutaneous tissue of the forearm [90]. Measurement of the NPD is useful in cases where sweat chloride measurements are equivocal or inconclusive, and genetic analysis shows *CFTR* mutations of unknown clinical significance [91]. The CF Foundation Therapeutics Development Network (CFF-TDN) has developed standardized procedures for recording NPD in order to reduce variability and improve consistency among NPD measurements in different centers [92]. In general, NPD measurements should be performed in both nostrils by properly trained personnel at experienced centers and the average of both readings should be recorded.

Chronic rhinosinusitis is common in patients with CF and is thought to be related to mucoviscidosis and nasal obstruction [93]. Interestingly, sinonasal polyposis also occurs frequently in patients with CF for unclear reasons. The prevalence of nasal and sinus polyps increases with age and has been shown to range between 6% and 48% in most series [94]. One possible explanation is that *CFTR* mutations including the ΔF508 mutation increase the risk for sinonasal polyposis. This is supported by the observation that *CFTR* mutations are common among the general population with chronic rhinosinusitis and nasal polyposis [95]. Moreover, such mutations also increase the risk of sinonasal anatomic abnormalities. For instance, patients homozygous for the ΔF508 mutation are far more likely to have frontal, maxillary or sphenoid sinus hypoplasia than the general population [96].

Pancreas

The degree of pancreatic insufficiency in patients with CF correlates well with the genotype (type of mutation) of *CFTR* [97]. *CFTR* dysfunction impairs the secretion of bicarbonate ions from pancreatic duct epithelial cells. Moreover, in a fashion similar to that in respiratory tract epithelia, proteinaceous secretions from the pancreas become viscid and desiccated. These secretions result in blockage of pancreatic ducts and acini with resultant inflammation. In most patients with CF, the pancreas is affected early in infancy and the pancreatic acini and ductules are filled with eosinophilic material [98]. Near total disruption of pancreatic parenchyma followed by replacement by fibrous tissue is seen in 85–90% of patients. Pancreatic calcifications on abdominal radiographs, typical of chronic pancreatitis, may be seen in some CF patients. As mentioned before, the term "cystic fibrosis" was coined for this disorder based on the presence of cysts and fibrotic areas within the pancreas in affected patients [5].

Pancreatic pathology in patients with CF is not limited to its exocrine elements. In CF patients with a severe phenotype, the islets of Langerhans become affected by the late second decade of life. Destruction of β-cells of the endocrine pancreas leads to progressive insulin deficiency, which manifests as impaired fasting glucose in initial stages and CF-related diabetes (CFRD) in end-stage pancreatic insufficiency [99]. For this reason, most experts advocate an oral glucose tolerance test (OGTT) for detection of subtle glycemic abnormalities. This approach may presumably allow earlier diagnosis of endocrine pancreatic insufficiency and treatment with insulin injections at this stage may retard decline in weight or pulmonary function [100]. However, to date, no randomized controlled trials have established the superiority of this approach over more conservative management strategies.

Intestines

Defective functioning of *CFTR* also affects the gastrointestinal epithelium. The basic pathophysiology is similar to that of the respiratory tract and results from impaired secretion of bicarbonate and chloride ions. Alteration of local pH and an ineffective mucus barrier lead to deranged innate immunity and promote small intestinal bacterial overgrowth [57]. Additionally, reduced secretion of bicarbonate ions lead to defective neutralization of gastric acid, denaturation of pancreatic enzymes and impaired formation of micelles [101]. Reduced intestinal motility and inspissated secretions can cause meconium ileus in the newborn [102], meconium plug syndrome in infants [103] and/or distal intestinal obstruction syndrome (DIOS) in older adults [104]. Malabsorption of macro- and micronutrients manifests as failure to thrive and can also result in vitamin deficiencies.

Liver and Gallbladder

Involvement of liver in patients with CF is uncommon in early life, but, may be found in up to 70% of adult CF patients [105]. Biliary cirrhosis is the hallmark lesion seen in patients with CF and develops secondary to blockage of intrahepatic bile ducts. In initial stages, focal biliary cirrhosis is evident, which progresses to multilobar biliary cirrhosis in later stages [106]. Histopathology of hepatic biopsy specimens demonstrates large, irregular parenchymal nodules with interspersed bands of fibrotic tissue. In some cases, fatty infiltration of hepatocytes may also occur [107].

Cholelithiasis is common in patients with CF and, in some cases, the gallbladder may undergo mucous metaplasia [108]. Hypoplasia of the gallbladder, atresia of the cystic duct and stenosis of the common bile duct are other lesions associated with CF [109].

Reproductive Tract

The reproductive tract is inevitably affected in all male patients with CF and more than 95% of such patients have infertility [110]. Infertility in such patients is attributable to azoospermia as sexual function is generally unimpaired. Inspissated secretions in the vas deferens, seminal vesicles and epididymis lead to atresia of these structures early in fetal life resulting in azoospermia. Inguinal hernia, hydrocele and undescended testes also occur more frequently in such patients [111]. Moreover, apart from CF, mutations in the *CFTR* gene have been associated with a distinct entity known as congenital absence of the vas deferens (CAVD) [112].

In girls with CF, mucus glands present in the cervix are distended with copious amounts of viscid mucus. Fertility rates are lower than the normal population and many patients experience secondary amenorrhea in adolescence, especially with pulmonary exacerbations [113].

Bones

As the life expectancy for patients with CF has increased over the past few years, bone disease has been recognized an increasingly common complication of the disease. Bone disease in such patients is a combined consequence of physical inactivity, vitamin D deficiency (due to malabsorption of fat-soluble vitamins), glucocorticoid therapy, altered sex hormone production and elevated levels of bone-active cytokines due to chronic inflammation [114]. Recent studies have shown that osteopenia is detectable in 85% of adult patients, whereas osteoporosis affects 10–34% of patients [115]. Interestingly, low bone mineral density (BMD) is observed even in patients who receive supplementation with usual doses (900 IU) of vitamin D [116].

Other Organ Systems

The full spectrum of pathology in CF patients is dependent on the genotype inherited and the effect of environmental factors and modifier genes [117]. Presence of *CFTR* on non-epithelial tissues has been recognized recently and the pleiotropic effects of *CFTR* have only been partially understood so far. Patients with CF also suffer from a variety of abnormalities relating to the neurologic, renal, endocrine and hematologic systems of the body [118, 119]. Some of these abnormalities, such as peripheral neuropathy, hemolytic anemia and bleeding diathesis, may attributable to deficiency of vitamins E and K. However, other abnormalities may be a manifestation of *CFTR* dysfunction [120].

Management

Management of patients with CF is best carried out by dedicated teams in specialized centers and involves education of patients and their families and use of non-pharmacologic and pharmacologic treatment modalities in conjunction with close monitoring and regular follow-ups. A multidisciplinary approach to management is necessary to ensure proper deployment of treatment modalities tailored to the individual needs of each patient and to maximize life expectancy while maintaining an optimum quality of life [121]. Before delving into the details of CF care, it would be useful to review the clinical features of this disease and discuss its differential diagnoses.

Clinical Features

Presentation of CF patients varies with the age of such patients and their underlying genotypic abnormalities [122]. Neonates and infants may present with meconium ileus, jaundice neonatorum, hypochloremic metabolic alkalosis and/or heat prostration. Toddlers and children may present with bulky, oily stools, cramping after feeding, excessive flatulence, sinonasal polyposis and/or rectal prolapse. Adolescents and adults may present with unexplained cirrhosis, acute pancreatitis, gallstones, recurrent respiratory tract infections or infection with atypical pathogens (such as *Staphylococcus aureus* or *Pseudomonas aeruginosa*).

In patients with CF, it is essential to obtain a complete history and perform a focused physical examination at each visit [123]. History taking should focus on eliciting symptoms of pulmonary exacerbation, gastrointestinal disturbance (esophagitis, constipation, flatulence), fat-soluble vitamin deficiencies (nyctalopia for vitamin A deficiency, bone pain and deformities for vitamin D deficiency, numbness/tingling for vitamin E deficiency and easy bruising for vitamin K deficiency), dietary history (calorie intake), adverse effects of treatment and adherence to medications. At the initial visit, a detailed family history is also indispensable; issues related to screening of CF and genetic counseling of parents are beyond the scope of this chapter [124]. Physical examination should include assessment of growth parameters (height and weight-for-age) and nutritional status (triceps skinfold thickness and wasted extremities), measurement of vital signs, general examination for presence of pallor, icterus or clubbing, inspection of nasal mucosa (inflamed turbinates and/or nasal polyps) and detailed pulmonary (wheezing indicative of bronchiolitis or crackles suggestive of bronchiectasis) and abdominal (hepatosplenomegaly, gut sounds, masses or rectal prolapse) examinations [125].

Differential Diagnosis

Diagnosis of CF requires the presence of laboratory evidence of *CFTR* dysfunction (elevated sweat chloride concentration, presence of two mutant *CFTR* alleles or characteristic NPD abnormalities) and disease-defining phenotypic features, such as sinonasal polyposis, chronic sinusitis, bronchiectasis, persistent pneumonia with characteristic CF pathogens (*Staphylococcus aureus*, *Pseudomonas aeruginosa* or other gram-negative rods), recurrent pancreatitis, exocrine pancreatic insufficiency, meconium ileus, fat-soluble vitamin deficiencies or obstructive azoospermia [78, 126]. A variety of other diseases may resemble the CF phenotype and therefore, the differential diagnosis of CF is broad. Celiac disease (and other malabsorptive disorders), asthma, recurrent pneumonia (and other pulmonary pathologies), immunodeficiency states and several other congenital disorders may be confused for CF [127].

Overview of Treatment

Optimal multidisciplinary care to CF patients can be provided through a coordinated network consisting of a pediatric pulmonologist, nurse specialist, physiotherapist and dietician. Components of care include prevention and prompt treatment of pulmonary exacerbations, salt supplementation, fat-soluble vitamin supplementation, zinc supplementation, pancreatic enzyme replacement, bronchodilator and mucolytic therapy coupled with pulmonary toilet and chest physiotherapy, assessment of bone health, endocrine evaluation and rehabilitative support [128]. Patient and family education is essential to help patients and their families cope with the stress of intensive medical management and promptly recognize complications. Psychosocial counseling is often required to help patients cope with the practical aspects of therapy and accommodate them in their lifestyle [129]. Dietician consultation is necessary to formulate a high-calorie, high-fat diet plan. Aerobic exercise and strength training have positive effects on quality of life and exercise programs for CF patients should be implemented (whenever possible) [130].

Treatment of Pulmonary Disease

Treatment of pulmonary disease in patients with CF involves bronchodilators (ipratropium), physical airway clearance (pulmonary toilet), airway rehydration therapies (hypertonic saline and/or mannitol), mucolytics (such as recombinant human DNAse), inhaled antibiotics and anti-inflammatory therapies. Avoidance of cigarette smoke exposure is essential; even passive smoking can adversely affect pulmonary function [131]. Bronchodilator therapy (with ipratropium or albuterol) is useful if patients have an element of airway hyperactivity [132]. Inhaled bronchodilators should be administered before chest physiotherapy to enhance pulmonary toilet.

Airway clearance should be done about four times a day at regular intervals to expectorate viscid secretions. Chest percussions delivered using a mechanical percussor are useful for postural drainage. Chest wall vibrators and airway oscillators are also frequently employed along with chest percussions to dislodge inspissated mucus from the smaller airways [133]. Directed cough maneuvers should be taught to patients to help efficiently expectorate loosed secretions and ensure optimal airway clearance [134].

Several other agents have been proven to enhance airway clearance by loosening airway mucus. Recombinant human DNAse administered daily in inhaled form can improve pulmonary function and reduce exacerbations [135]. Airway hydration therapies including inhaled hypertonic saline (7%) and inhaled mannitol can provide additional clinical benefit and have been shown to produce sustained improvement in pulmonary function [136]. Use of corticosteroids is more controversial, but generally, inhaled corticosteroids have not been shown to improve long-term outcomes [137]. A short course of systemic corticosteroids may be used in patients who develop acute pulmonary exacerbation. However, administration of prolonged courses of systemic corticosteroids can lead to adverse effects and overall worse outcome; therefore, long-term therapy with systemic steroids should be avoided [138]. Use of ibuprofen in patients under the age of 13 years can reduce pulmonary inflammation and slow decline of FEV_1 [139]. Prophylactic azithromycin has also been proven to reduce the decline in FEV_1 due to its dual antimicrobial and anti-inflammatory properties [140].

Prompt recognition of pulmonary exacerbations is essential to institute empiric antimicrobial therapy and prevent decline in pulmonary function [141, 142]. Signs of pulmonary exacerbation in patients with CF include a change in the quantity or quality of sputum, new-onset hemoptysis or increase in quantity, worsening dyspnea or cough, generalized fatigue/malaise, fever, change in sinus discharge, change in pulmonary examination, acute decrease in FEV_1 of $\geq$ 10% and/or a new infiltrate on chest radiographs [143]. Patients with evidence of acute pulmonary exacerbation should be treated with antimicrobial therapy (either inhaled, oral or intravenous). In patients who are on prophylactic antibiotics, a change in antibiotics is advisable to help eradicate infection [144]. Patients with a mild pulmonary exacerbation may be treated with oral antibiotics, whereas patients with a severe pulmonary exacerbation, multidrug resistant pathogens or exacerbation refractory to oral antibiotics should be treated with intravenous antibiotics. The optimal duration of treatment for acute pulmonary exacerbations is 7–14 days [145]. However, it is important to exclude allergic bronchopulmonary mycoses and/or non-tuberculous mycobacterial infections in such patients. Allergic pulmonary mycoses are treated with a combination of steroids and anti-fungal agents, while non-tuberculous mycobacterial infections are treated with multiple antibiotics for 6 months [146, 147].

Choice of antibiotic therapy in CF patients with acute pulmonary exacerbation should be guided by sputum cultures (whenever possible) [148]. Empiric therapy can be instituted with systemic antibiotics, such as aminoglycosides, penicillins, cephalosporins, macrolides, sulfamethoxazole–trimethoprim, ciprofloxacin, or other systemic antibiotics [149]. As patients with CF often develop colonization with bacteria, the goal of antibiotic therapy is to suppress bacterial load to a level where symptoms are minimal. The optimal choice of antibiotic therapy differs according to the microorganism cultured. *Hemophilus influenzae* can usually be eradicated completely by therapy with penicillins (such as amoxicillin–clavulanic acid) or cephalosporins (such as cefixime) [150]. *Staphylococcus aureus* (methicillin-sensitive) can be treated with cloxacillin, cephalexin, cefazolin, amoxicillin–clavulanic acid, or a macrolide [151]. Methicillin-resistant *Staphylococcus aureus* (MRSA) should be treated aggressively with vancomycin, linezolid or other antibiotics as MRSA infection has been associated with a rapid decline in pulmonary infection [152]. *Pseudomonas aeruginosa* is notorious for colonizing lungs of CF patients; however, evidence supports the concept that early, aggressive treatment of *Pseudomonas aeruginosa* infections can delay, or even prevent, colonization with this deadly organism [153]. For treating acute pulmonary exacerbations due to this organism, a combination of tobramycin and either an antipseudomonal β-lactam or ciprofloxacin should be used. In case of tobramycin resistance, amikacin can be used. Inhaled tobramycin is often used in patients with mild infections due to *Pseudomonas aeruginosa*. Following treatment of the initial infection, chronic suppressive therapy with inhaled gentamycin, tobramycin or colistin should be employed [154]. For patients with suspected *Mycoplasma* or *Chlamydia* infections, a macrolide is the agent of choice. In later stages of the disease, patients may develop infections with multidrug resistant organisms, such as *Burkholderia cenocepacia*, *Stenotrophomonas maltophilia* or *Achromobacter xylosoxidans* [155, 156]. Patients with *Stenotrophomonas maltophilia* infection may be treated with a quinolone, aminoglycoside or sulfamethoxazole–trimethoprim. For *Achromobacter xylosoxidans* infections, similar agents (quinolone, aminoglycoside, sulfamethoxazole–trimethoprim or cefepime) may be effective. *Burkholderia cenocepacia* infections are the most difficult to treat and often require administration of triple intravenous antibiotics (tobramycin, meropenem and ceftazidime or sulfamethoxazole–trimethoprim) [157]. In some cases, this organism may be sensitive to doxycycline, in which case it may be used. Generally, *Burkholderia cenocepacia* infections have a poor prognosis and indicate end-stage pulmonary disease [158].

Other supportive therapies for management of pulmonary disease include oxygen therapy, non-invasive positive pressure ventilation (NIPPV), mechanical ventilation and endoscopic procedures. Oxygen therapy and NIPPV is usually required in advanced pulmonary disease in order to maintain oxygen saturation and prevent the development of cor pulmonale [159]. In some patients with acute respiratory failure, mechanical ventilation may be necessary and such issues should ideally be discussed with patients before such a situation arises. Fiberoptic bronchoscopy has been used to perform bronchopulmonary lavage with instillation of antibiotic and mucolytic agents in patients with atelectasis secondary to mucus impaction [160]. However, there is no evidence currently available to prove that such interventions provide any meaningful long-term benefit.

Some CF patients may develop complications of pulmonary disease such as a pneumothorax or massive hemoptysis (due to erosion of a bronchial vessel). Management of such patients may require consultation with a thoracic surgeon and/or interventional radiologist. Pleurodesis may be necessary for patients with recurrent pneumothorax after initial chest tube placement [161]. However, this mode of therapy might have a negative impact on eligibility for lung transplantation and thus it should only be resorted to if other measures fail to control recurrent pneumothoraces. For patients with massive hemoptysis, bronchial artery angioembolization or lobectomy may be needed in rare cases [162]. In carefully selected patients, lung transplantation may be a feasible option to prolong survival and improve quality of life [163].

Treatment of Gastrointestinal Disease

As mentioned in the section on pathophysiology, patients with CF have multiple defects in digestion and absorption of nutrients. A dietician evaluation for the formulation of a high-fiber, high-fat, high-calorie diet plan is necessary in most patients [164]. Pancreatic enzyme replacement is inevitable in patients with exocrine pancreatic insufficiency. Fat-soluble vitamins and zinc supplementation should be offered to all patients. In patients with bile or gastric acid reflux, proton pump inhibitors (or histaminergic receptor blockers) can be used [165]. As intestinal motility is often reduced, polyethylene glycol and a high-fiber diet are necessary to prevent constipation and/or the development of DIOS [166]. In patients with impending DIOS, Gastrografin enema may be a useful option for bowel cleansing.

Treatment of Endocrine Abnormalities

Patients with CF (older than 10 years of age) should be regularly screened using OGTT for the development of endocrine pancreatic insufficiency [167]. In patients who develop impaired glucose tolerance, treatment with once-daily insulin injections may be instituted (based on expert opinion) [168]. Safety of oral hypoglycemic agents in patients with CFRD has not been established. Theoretically, use of insulin injections seems intuitive as progressive insulin deficiency is an expected consequence of the natural course of the disease. Moreover, onset of CFRD in patients has been associated with a worse outcome and early institution of insulin replacement may thus be beneficial [169].

Bone health in patients with CF is adversely affected and calcium and vitamin D supplementation should be routinely offered. In patients with osteoporosis and/or osteopenia, bisphosphonate therapy may be offered, although bisphosphonates do not reduce the long-term risk of fractures [170]. Delayed puberty and short stature are also common complaints in CF patients and are direct consequences of sex hormone abnormalities and nutritional deficiencies [171]. Endocrinology referral should be encouraged for such patients as some patients may benefit from timely hormone replacement therapy [172].

Other Aspects of Treatment

Patients with sino-pulmonary disease often require topical steroid sprays and nasal rinses along with antibiotic courses for episodes of acute bacterial rhinosinusitis. In patients with extensive chronic rhinosinusitis, functional endoscopic sinus surgery may be necessary to remove polyps, relieve sinus obstruction and restore normal sinus function [173].

As all patients with CF lose a substantial amount of sodium chloride in sweat, patients should be educated regarding the symptoms of salt depletion [174]. Pediatric patients usually require salt supplementation, while older patients may be advised to increase the amount of salt in their diet as needed.

As the life expectancy for CF patients improves, advanced reproductive technologies have gained more importance. Men with CF should be offered epididymal aspiration for sperm retrieval [175], which may allow these patients to father children through *in vitro* fertilization.

Medical care for CF patients represents a significant financial and time burden for patients and their families. Consequently, the prevalence of depression among CF patients is higher than that of the normal population [176]. Such patients require continuous psychosocial counseling and support. Palliative and end-of-life care for patients with advanced disease should be discussed with patients and their families and advanced directives should be planned ahead of time [177].

Novel Treatment Strategies

Conventional approaches to management of CF patients have focused on treating the complications of *CFTR* dysfunction. However, novel approaches to CF treatment go a step ahead and focus on correcting the gene defect that leads to the pleiotropic manifestations of CF phenotype. Most of these novel strategies to treat CF are still in their incipient stages; however, they hold immense promise in that they may eventually help to find a definitive way to cure CF [178].

Gene therapy for CF was once an area of intensive research, but, favorable results have not been achieved in clinical studies [179]. The principle underlying gene therapy is to deliver normal *CFTR* genes into CF affected cells through the use of a viral vector (often adenovirus). Transfer of normal *CFTR* genes into affected cells may allow normal expression of *CFTR* channels and ameliorate the phenotype features of the disease. However, to date, no definitive method of gene delivery has been perfected and results in clinical trials and studies have been variable and inconsistent [180]. Use of adeno-associated virus (AAV) vectors, lipid-based gene transfer vectors, compacted DNA nanoparticles and CpG-depleted DNA motifs have been tried without much success [181, 182]. Concerns regarding the long-term safety of such preparations have also been raised. Therefore, at present, gene therapy does not seem to be a feasible therapeutic strategy.

Over the past decade, CF research has seen a paradigm shift from gene therapy to the development of small molecules capable of addressing the functional *CFTR* defects at the protein level [183]. Such a treatment strategy is grounded in the principles of precision medicine and aims to tailor medications to the precise defects in protein biosynthesis or mutant protein function [178]. As mentioned in the section on pathophysiology, different classes of *CFTR* gene mutations lead to *CFTR* dysfunction through different mechanisms. For instance, patients with G551D mutation have defects in

CFTR channel gating [64]. Small molecules capable of potentiating cAMP-mediated *CFTR* activation have been developed through the use of high-throughput screening [184]. Ivacaftor (previously known as VX-770) is an example of such a *CFTR potentiator* and has recently been approved by the FDA for use in patients with the G551D gating mutation. Results of clinical trials evaluating the efficacy of this molecule have shown favorable outcomes, which are comparable to that achieved with conventional treatment options [185]. Likewise, lumacaftor (VX-809) is an example of a *CFTR corrector*—a small molecule that can correct the processing of mutant *CFTR* polypeptide and increase its expression on the cell membrane [180]. In the TRAFFIC and TRANSPORT trials, ivacaftor–lumacaftor combination therapy showed promising results in CF patients who were homozygous for the ΔF508 mutation [187].

Development of small molecules that target each step of *CFTR* biosynthesis and cellular processing holds immense promise for improving outcomes of CF patients. Experimental studies have shown that treatment of CF-affected cells with histone deacetylase (HDAC) inhibitors and silencers of small interfering ribonucleic acid (siRNA) can increase cellular expression of ΔF508 mutant *CFTR* [188, 189]. For patients with class V (mis-splicing) mutations, use of specific antisense oligonucleotides is being explored [190]. Likewise, in patients with premature stop codons, use of small molecules (such as ataluren) to induce translational read-through of premature stop codons is being evaluated in certain clinical trials [191]. These novel treatment modalities are still in experimental stages and their cost-effectiveness and widespread availability needs to be improved [192, 193]. However, development of personalized medications that aim to precisely correct *CFTR* defects at the protein level holds the key to finding a definitive cure for CF in the future.

Outcome Measures

As novel treatment strategies for CF are being developed, the need for having accurate and valid outcome measures has become more important than ever. Traditionally, pulmonary function tests and imaging-based outcome measures have been used to assess disease severity and effect of drugs. With the development of drugs that correct *CFTR* function at an early age, novel outcome measures and sensitive biomarkers have been explored [194].

Pulmonary Function Testing

A number of parameters derived from pulmonary function tests have been used to assess the effect of drugs in clinical trials. Conventionally used parameters included FEV_1 (i.e., the forced expiratory volume in one second), forced vital capacity (FVC) and the ratio of FEV_1 to FVC [195]. Newer parameters that have been evaluated include maximum mid-expiratory flow ($FEF_{25-75\%}$) and flow when 75% of FVC has been exhaled ($FEF_{75\%}$) [196]. While these parameters are useful for assessing the effect of drugs and have some prognostic significance, their utility is limited by the fact that they are deranged late in pulmonary disease and spirometry cannot be reliably performed in children below the age of 6 years.

For infants and young children, infant pulmonary function testing has become possible through the use of the raised volume rapid thoracoabdominal compression (RVRTC) technique [197]. Clinical studies using RVRTC have demonstrated that pulmonary function may be affected as early as 3 months of life in CF patients [198]. Availability of standardized guidelines and commercial kits has enabled the use of RVRTC as an endpoint in clinical trials. However, RVRTC-based infant pulmonary function testing is still limited to centers experienced in the use of this technique [194].

Another method of assessing pulmonary function in young children with CF is through the use of multiple breath washout (MBW) tests [199]. This method of testing provides two useful measures viz. functional residual capacity (FRC) and lung clearance index (LCI). LCI measures ventilation inhomogeneity by determining the washout of an inert gas during normal breathing and is an indirect indicator of small airway disease [200]. Clinical studies have shown that LCI is superior to standard spirometry for the detection of early lung disease [201]. LCI has also been demonstrated to correlate well with structural lung damage as noted on thoracic computed tomography (CT) scans [202]. Moreover, MBW has been shown to be equivalent to RVRTC for detecting lung disease in infants [203]. The only drawback of using LCI is that it requires expensive equipment and may need sedation in infants.

Imaging-Based Measures

Multiple imaging modalities have been used for the evaluation of CF-associated lung damage. The most commonly used modality for assessing bronchiectasis in patients with CF is high-resolution CT. Clinical studies have shown that CT scans are more sensitive in detecting lung disease than spirometry [204]. However, lung damage detected on CT scans correlates weakly with functional parameters. Different CT-based scoring systems have also been developed and validated [205]. As an example, the CT scan bronchiectasis score (Brody-II system) has been shown to be a predictor of pulmonary exacerbation rate [206]. The major disadvantage of this imaging modality is the significant radiation burden that it entails. On average, the radiation exposure from a single CT chest scan is equivalent to that from about 200–400 plain chest radiographs [207].

Pulmonary magnetic resonance imaging (MRI) has been explored as a diagnostic tool in research studies. Initially, the utility of MRI for pulmonary imaging was limited by motion artifacts and signal interference from extra-pulmonary tissues. Technical advances in the field of radiology have overcome some of these limitations and have enabled the use of MRI for obtaining images of airway and pulmonary parenchyma [208]. MRI-based scoring systems are being developed to standardize and quantify the degree of lung damage on MRI scans. The major advantage of MRI is the ability to acquire images of the pulmonary parenchyma that are almost equivalent in quality to that of CT without any associated radiation burden. However, the use of MRI is limited in clinical practice by the fact that MRI has a considerably long acquisition time (~30 min) for which sedation is nearly always necessary and MRI is less sensitive for detecting pathology of smaller airways [209].

^{18}Fluorodeoxyglucose (^{18}FDG) positron emission tomography (PET) is a functional imaging modality that generates images of the pulmonary parenchyma based on the uptake of radioisotope. Areas of active inflammation and infection demonstrate avid uptake of ^{18}FDG and show up as bright areas on PET scanning. In order to map spots of radiotracer uptake to anatomical areas, FDG-PET/CT scans are performed and provide more information than CT scanning alone [210]. However, routine use of FDG-PET/CT scans in CF patients has not been adopted yet in clinical practice or as primary end-points in randomized clinical trials.

Sputum Biomarkers

Sputum can be readily obtained in most children with CF who are aged 10 years or above. A number of sputum biomarkers have been evaluated in observational studies and shown to have good validity for assessment of pulmonary inflammation and/or infection. Sputum neutrophil count, neutrophil elastase activity and IL-8 concentration have been shown to have a good correlation with disease severity scores and overall quality of health measures [211, 212]. Further clinical studies are currently underway to assess other sputum characteristics, such as sputum dry weight, sputum rheology, biochemical composition, surface tension and impedance.

Blood-Based Biomarkers

Despite their potential, blood-based and serum biomarkers have not been widely used in clinical trials of CF. Observational studies to date have evaluated more than 70 circulating biomarkers of CF disease activity [213]. Acute phase proteins, such as C-reactive protein (CRP), serum amyloid A (SAA) and neutrophil elastase antiprotease complex, have been found to correlate well with disease exacerbations [214, 215]. Of these, CRP is the most widely studied biomarker and can be useful as a marker of pulmonary exacerbation [213]. CRP also holds promise to be used as an endpoint in randomized clinical trials.

Potential Difference

As discussed in the section on pathophysiology, NPD is an indirect measure of *CFTR* dysfunction and has been used in various clinical trials as an endpoint. Clinical studies have shown that NPD correlates well with the number and severity of *CFTR* gene mutations [194]. CFF-TDN has developed standardized procedures for recording NPD in order to reduce variability and improve consistency among NPD measurements in different centers [92]. In addition to NPD, potential difference measurements can also be obtained from the lower airways using fiberoptic bronchoscopy [216]. Usually, such measurements are obtained in clinical trials of gene therapy or inhaled drugs, where only the pulmonary tissues are affected by the treatment. Intestinal current measurement (ICM) is based on the same basic principle as NPD and provides a useful way of assessing pancreatic involvement in CF patients [217]. As is the case for NPD, guidelines have been formulated by CCF-TDN for standardization of ICM.

Sweat Chloride Test

Sweat chloride testing is a cornerstone for diagnosis of CF and has been in use for over four decades in research and clinical practice. Sweat chloride directly correlates with *CFTR* function in a dose-effect manner and is a sensitive indicator of *CFTR* dysfunction [218]. Pilocarpine-induced iontophoresis is a useful method for determining the concentration of sweat chloride and standardization of measurements makes it feasible for use in multicenter trials [220]. This method of testing is least invasive and does not carry a risk of any significant complications. Due to these advantages, sweat chloride testing is the most commonly employed endpoint in clinical trials.

Prognosis and Risk Factors

As CF is a hereditary disorder, the prime risk factor for the development of this disease is the inheritance of two mutant alleles. Being an autosomal recessive disorder, the risk of CF in a newborn child born to carrier parents is 1 in 4. A family history of CF can significantly increase the risk of CF as the diagnosis of this disorder in a family member implies the presence of carriers in the pedigree. All newborns in the United States are screened for CF with an immunoreactive trypsinogen test [220]. Results of two randomized clinical trials suggest that the implementation of neonatal screening improves clinical outcomes and is highly cost-effective [221].

In patients diagnosed with CF, a number of factors can affect long-term prognosis. Genotype (i.e., the class of mutation) is an important prognostic factor; for instance, patients with the ΔF508 mutation generally have a worse prognosis [222]. Conversely, patients with a class V mutation have a better prognosis. Gender has been established to be a prognostic factor with female patients generally having an overall worse prognosis [16]. This observation may be attributable to hormonal differences and propensity to recurrent respiratory infections [17]. Decline in pulmonary function as reflected by a decrease in FEV_1, FEV_1/FVC ratio, $FEF_{25-75\%}$ or $FEF_{75\%}$ is associated with worse prognosis [195]. Sweat chloride concentration correlates directly with CFTR dysfunction and higher sweat chloride concentration at diagnosis is an indicator of poor prognosis [223]. Microbial colonization of lungs in CF patients with certain organisms portends a worse prognosis. In particular, colonization with *Pseudomonas aeruginosa*, MSSA or both is associated with a rapid decline in pulmonary function and an overall worse outcome [224].

Organisms belonging to the *Burkholderia cepacia* complex, especially *Burkholderia cenocepacia*, are the most difficult to treat and are associated with the worst outcome [158]. Development of exocrine pancreatic insufficiency and CFRD are both associated with worse prognosis in patients with CF [97, 169]. Clinical studies have shown that development of pancreatic insufficiency is associated with a rapid decline in pulmonary function and increased risk of mortality [225]. CF-related liver disease is another complication of CF that is becoming more common with increased life expectancy. As per current literature, CF-related liver disease is the third most common cause of death in CF patients with first two being pulmonary exacerbation and transplant-related complications [226]. Development of CF-related liver disease is a marker of severe disease with an estimated mortality rate of 2.5%.

CF is a multisystem disorder that limits life expectancy, though survival rates have tremendously improved over the past few decades as a consequence of improved medical care [10]. The median cumulative survival for patients with CF is now 37 years in the US and will continue to improve further in the coming years. The most common cause of death continues to be end-stage lung disease and decline in pulmonary function is the prime life-limiting factor [227]. Children early in life often have recurrent respiratory infections, but, multidisciplinary care in specialized care centers can allow them to continue their normal activities and complete their education. Increased life expectancy, however, brings with it complex psychosocial issues relating to social relationships, reproductive health, mood disorders, substance abuse and financial burden [228]. In the modern era, patients with CF can find employment and live a married life.

Conclusion

CF is an autosomal recessive multisystem disorder that results from a genetic defect in *CFTR* gene and occurs in 1 in 2,500 childbirths in the Caucasian population. Being a pleiotropic gene, *CFTR* dysfunction manifests as bronchiectasis, recurrent pneumonia, sinonasal polyposis, pancreatic insufficiency, fat-soluble vitamin deficiencies, diabetes mellitus, infertility and other systemic abnormalities. Management of the disease includes prompt recognition and treatment of pulmonary exacerbations, chest physiotherapy and pulmonary toilet, bronchodilators, mucolytics, airway hydration therapies, nutritional support, mineral and vitamin supplementation, pancreatic enzyme replacement, screening for diabetes mellitus and hormone replacement (if needed). CF is a life-limiting disorder, although the life expectancy for patients is improving and currently stands at 37 years in the United States. With continuous psychosocial support, comprehensive medical care and vocational training, individuals can cope well with the stress of their illness and live a productive life.

Conflict of Interests

The authors have no conflict of interests to disclose.

References

[1] Strausbaugh, S.D., Davis, P. B. (2007). Cystic fibrosis: a review of epidemiology and pathobiology. *Clinics in Chest Medicine*, *28*(2), 279-288.

[2] Mornon, J. P., Lehn, P. and Callebaut, I. (2009). Molecular models of the open and closed states of the whole human CFTR protein. *Cellular and Molecular Life Sciences*, *66*(21), 3469-3486.

[3] Farrell, P. M. (2008). The prevalence of cystic fibrosis in the European Union. *Journal of Cystic Fibrosis*, *7*(5), 450-453.

[4] Davis, P. B. (2006). Cystic fibrosis since 1938. *American Journal of Respiratory and Critical Care Medicine*, *173*(5), 475-482.

[5] Sheppard, M. N. and Nicholson, A. G. (2002). The pathology of cystic fibrosis. *Current Diagnostic Pathology*, *8*(1), 50-59.

[6] Lyczak, J. B., Cannon, C. L. and Pier, G. B. (2002). Lung infections associated with cystic fibrosis. *Clinical Microbiology Reviews*, *15*(2), 194-222.

[7] Rogers, C. S., Stoltz, D. A., Meyerholz, D. K., Ostedgaard, L. S., Rokhlina, T., Taft, P. J., et al. (2008). Disruption of the CFTR gene produces a model of cystic fibrosis in newborn pigs. *Science*, *321*(5897), 1837-1841.

[8] Fanen, P., Wohlhuter-Haddad, A. and Hinzpeter, A. (2014). Genetics of cystic fibrosis: CFTR mutation classifications toward genotype-based CF therapies. *The International Journal of Biochemistry and Cell Biology*, *52*, 94-102.

[9] The Cystic Fibrosis Genetic Analysis Consortium. (2016). *Cystic Fibrosis Mutation Database*. The Hospital for Sick Children (Toronto). URL: http://www.genet.sickkids.on.ca/ (Last accessed 11th March, 2016).

[10] Dodge, J. A., Lewis, P. A., Stanton, M. and Wilsher, J. (2007). Cystic fibrosis mortality and survival in the UK: 1947–2003. *European Respiratory Journal*, *29*(3), 522-526.

[11] Farrell, P., Joffe, S., Foley, L., Canny, G. J., Mayne, P. and Rosenberg, M. (2007). Diagnosis of cystic fibrosis in the Republic of Ireland: epidemiology and costs. *Irish Medical Journal*, *100*(8), 557.

[12] Spoonhower, K. A. and Davis, P. B. (2016). Epidemiology of Cystic Fibrosis. *Clinics in Chest Medicine*, *37*(1), 1-8.

[13] Bowler, I. M., Estlin, E. J. and Littlewood, J. M. (1993). Cystic fibrosis in Asians. *Archives of Disease in Childhood*, *68*(1), 120-122.

[14] Bobadilla, J. L., Macek, M., Fine, J. P. and Farrell, P. M. (2002). Cystic fibrosis: a worldwide analysis of CFTR mutations—correlation with incidence data and application to screening. *Human Mutation*, *19*(6), 575-606.

[15] Alfonso-Sánchez, M. A., Pérez-Miranda, A. M., García-Obregón, S. and Peña, J. A. (2010). An evolutionary approach to the high frequency of the Delta F508 CFTR mutation in European populations. *Medical Hypotheses*, *74*(6), 989-992.

[16] Nick, J. A., Chacon, C. S., Brayshaw, S. J., Jones, M. C., Barboa, C. M., Clair, C. G. S., et al. (2010). Effects of gender and age at diagnosis on disease progression in long-term survivors of cystic fibrosis. *American Journal of Respiratory and Critical Care Medicine*, *182*(5), 614-626.

[17] Carey, M. A., Card, J. W., Voltz, J. W., Germolec, D. R., Korach, K. S. and Zeldin, D. C. (2007). The impact of sex and sex hormones on lung physiology and disease: lessons from animal studies. *American Journal of Physiology-Lung Cellular and Molecular Physiology*, *293*(2), L272-L278.

[18] O'Connor, G. T., Quinton, H. B., Kneeland, T., Kahn, R., Lever, T., Maddock, J., et al. (2003). Median household income and mortality rate in cystic fibrosis. *Pediatrics*, *111*(4), e333-e339.

[19] Schechter, M. S., Shelton, B. J., Margolis, P. A. and FitzSimmons, S. C. (2001). The association of socioeconomic status with outcomes in cystic

fibrosis patients in the United States. *American Journal of Respiratory and Critical Care Medicine*, *163*(6), 1331-1337.

[20] Kulich, M., Rosenfeld, M., Goss, C. H. and Wilmott, R. (2003). Improved survival among young patients with cystic fibrosis. *The Journal of Pediatrics*, *142*(6), 631-636.

[21] Parker-McGill, K., Nugent, M., Bersie, R., Hoffman, G., Rock, M., Baker, M., et al. (2015). Changing incidence of cystic fibrosis in Wisconsin, USA. *Pediatric Pulmonology*, *50*(11), 1065-1072.

[22] Lai, H. J., Cheng, Y. and Farrell, P. M. (2005). The survival advantage of patients with cystic fibrosis diagnosed through neonatal screening: evidence from the United States Cystic Fibrosis Foundation registry data. *The Journal of Pediatrics*, *147*(3), S57-S63.

[23] Castellani, C., Picci, L., Tamanini, A., Girardi, P., Rizzotti, P. and Assael, B. M. (2009). Association between carrier screening and incidence of cystic fibrosis. *JAMA*, *302*(23), 2573-2579.

[24] Berdiev, B. K., Qadri, Y. J. and Benos, D. J. (2009). Assessment of the CFTR and ENaC association. *Molecular BioSystems*, *5*(2), 123-127.

[25] McCarthy, V. A. and Harris, A. (2005). The CFTR gene and regulation of its expression. *Pediatric Pulmonology*, *40*(1), 1-8.

[26] Koh, J., Sferra, T. J. and Collins, F. S. (1993). Characterization of the cystic fibrosis transmembrane conductance regulator promoter region. Chromatin context and tissue-specificity. *Journal of Biological Chemistry*, *268*(21), 15912-15921.

[27] Bienvenu, T., Lacronique, V., Raymondjean, M., Cazeneuve, C., Hubert, D., Kaplan, J. C. and Beldjord, C. (1995). Three novel sequence variations in the 5′ upstream region of the cystic fibrosis transmembrane conductance regulator (CFTR) gene: two polymorphisms and one putative molecular defect. *Human Genetics*, *95*(6), 698-702.

[28] Bartoszewski, R., Rab, A., Twitty, G., Stevenson, L., Fortenberry, J., Piotrowski, A., et al. (2008). The mechanism of cystic fibrosis transmembrane conductance regulator transcriptional repression during the unfolded protein response. *Journal of Biological Chemistry*, *283*(18), 12154-12165.

[29] Montrose-Rafizadeh, C., Blackmon, D. L., Hamosh, A., Oliva, M. M., Hawkins, A. L., Curristin, S. M., et al. (1992). Regulation of cystic fibrosis transmembrane conductance regulator (CFTR) gene transcription and alternative RNA splicing in a model of developing

intestinal epithelium. *Journal of Biological Chemistry*, *267*(27), 19299-19305.

[30] Rowntree, R. and Harris, A. (2002). DNA polymorphisms in potential regulatory elements of the CFTR gene alter transcription factor binding. *Human Genetics*, *111*(1), 66-74.

[31] Ramalho, A. S., Beck, S., Meyer, M., Penque, D., Cutting, G. R. and Amaral, M. D. (2002). Five percent of normal cystic fibrosis transmembrane conductance regulator mRNA ameliorates the severity of pulmonary disease in cystic fibrosis. *American Journal of Respiratory Cell and Molecular Biology*, *27*(5), 619-627.

[32] Pittman, N., Shue, G., Neal, S. L. and Walsh, M. J. (1995). Transcription of cystic fibrosis transmembrane conductance regulator requires a CCAAT-like element for both basal and cAMP-mediated regulation. *Journal of Biological Chemistry*, *270*(48), 28848-28857.

[33] Gillen, A. E., Gosalia, N., Leir, S. H. and Harris, A. (2011). MicroRNA regulation of expression of the cystic fibrosis transmembrane conductance regulator gene. *Biochemical Journal*, *438*(1), 25-32.

[34] Amaral, M. D. (2005). Processing of CFTR: traversing the cellular maze—how much CFTR needs to go through to avoid cystic fibrosis? *Pediatric Pulmonology*, *39*(6), 479-491.

[35] Amaral, M. D. (2004). CFTR and chaperones. *Journal of Molecular Neuroscience*, *23*(1-2), 41-48.

[36] Qu, B. H. and Thomas, P. J. (1996). Alteration of the Cystic Fibrosis Transmembrane Conductance Regulator Folding Pathway: Effects of the ΔF508 mutation on the thermodynamic stability and folding yield of NBD1. *Journal of Biological Chemistry*, *271*(13), 7261-7264.

[37] Jensen, T. J., Loo, M. A., Pind, S., Williams, D. B., Goldberg, A. L. and Riordan, J. R. (1995). Multiple proteolytic systems, including the proteasome, contribute to CFTR processing. *Cell*, *83*(1), 129-135.

[38] Ward, C. L., Omura, S. and Kopito, R. R. (1995). Degradation of CFTR by the ubiquitin-proteasome pathway. *Cell*, *83*(1), 121-127.

[39] Ellgaard, L. and Helenius, A. (2003). Quality control in the endoplasmic reticulum. *Nature Reviews Molecular Cell Biology*, *4*(3), 181-191.

[40] Yoo, J. S., Moyer, B. D., Bannykh, S., Yoo, H. M., Riordan, J. R. and Balch, W. E. (2002). Non-conventional trafficking of the cystic fibrosis transmembrane conductance regulator through the early secretory pathway. *Journal of Biological Chemistry*, *277*(13), 11401-11409.

[41] Li, C. and Naren, A. P. (2005). Macromolecular complexes of cystic fibrosis transmembrane conductance regulator and its interacting partners. *Pharmacology and Therapeutics*, *108*(2), 208-223.

[42] Rogan, M. P., Stoltz, D. A. and Hornick, D. B. (2011). Cystic fibrosis transmembrane conductance regulator intracellular processing, trafficking, and opportunities for mutation-specific treatment. *Chest Journal*, *139*(6), 1480-1490.

[43] Akabas, M. H. (2000). Cystic fibrosis transmembrane conductance regulator structure and function of an epithelial chloride channel. Journal of Biological Chemistry, 275(6), 3729-3732.

[44] Sun, F., Hug, M. J., Bradbury, N. A. and Frizzell, R. A. (2000). Protein kinase A associates with cystic fibrosis transmembrane conductance regulator via an interaction with ezrin. *Journal of Biological Chemistry*, *275*(19), 14360-14366.

[45] Sharma, M., Benharouga, M., Hu, W. and Lukacs, G. L. (2001). Conformational and temperature-sensitive stability defects of the ΔF508 cystic fibrosis transmembrane conductance regulator in post-endoplasmic reticulum compartments. *Journal of Biological Chemistry*, *276*(12), 8942-8950.

[46] Riordan, J. R. (1993). The cystic fibrosis transmembrane conductance regulator. *Annual Review of Physiology*, *55*(1), 609-630.

[47] Tarran, R., Grubb, B. R., Gatzy, J. T., Davis, C. W. and Boucher, R. C. (2001). The relative roles of passive surface forces and active ion transport in the modulation of airway surface liquid volume and composition. *The Journal of General Physiology*, *118*(2), 223-236.

[48] Novak, I., Wang, J., Henriksen, K. L., Haanes, K. A., Krabbe, S., Nitschke, R. and Hede, S. E. (2011). Pancreatic bicarbonate secretion involves two proton pumps. *Journal of Biological Chemistry*, *286*(1), 280-289.

[49] Quinton, P. M. (2010). Role of epithelial $HCO3^-$ transport in mucin secretion: lessons from cystic fibrosis. *American Journal of Physiology-Cell Physiology*, *299*(6), C1222-C1233.

[50] Borowitz, D. (2015). CFTR, bicarbonate, and the pathophysiology of cystic fibrosis. *Pediatric Pulmonology*, *50*(S40), S24-S30.

[51] Thornton, D. J., Rousseau, K. and McGuckin, M. A. (2008). Structure and function of the polymeric mucins in airways mucus. *Annual Review of Physiology*, *70*, 459-486.

[52] Tarran, R. (2004). Regulation of airway surface liquid volume and mucus transport by active ion transport. *Proceedings of the American Thoracic Society*, *1*(1), 42-46.

[53] Mall, M. A. (2008). Role of cilia, mucus, and airway surface liquid in mucociliary dysfunction: lessons from mouse models. *Journal of Aerosol Medicine and Pulmonary Drug Delivery*, *21*(1), 13-24.

[54] Pezzulo, A. A., Tang, X. X., Hoegger, M. J., Alaiwa, M. H. A., Ramachandran, S., Moninger, T. O., et al. (2012). Reduced airway surface pH impairs bacterial killing in the porcine cystic fibrosis lung. *Nature*, *487*(7405), 109-113.

[55] Sayeed, S., Nistico, L., St Croix, C. and Di, Y. P. (2013). Multifunctional role of human SPLUNC1 in Pseudomonas aeruginosa infection. *Infection and Immunity*, *81*(1), 285-291.

[56] Lynch, S. V. and Bruce, K. D. (2013). The cystic fibrosis airway microbiome. *Cold Spring Harbor Perspectives in Medicine*, *3*(3), a009738.

[57] Gelfond, D. and Borowitz, D. (2013). Gastrointestinal complications of cystic fibrosis. *Clinical Gastroenterology and Hepatology*, *11*(4), 333-342.

[58] Van de Weert–van Leeuwen, P. B., Van Meegen, M. A., Speirs, J. J., Pals, D. J., Rooijakkers, S. H., Van der Ent, C. K., et al. (2013). Optimal complement-mediated phagocytosis of *Pseudomonas aeruginosa* by monocytes is Cystic Fibrosis Transmembrane Conductance Regulator–dependent. *American Journal of Respiratory Cell and Molecular Biology*, *49*(3), 463-470.

[59] Mickle, J. E. and Cutting, G. R. (2000). Genotype-phenotype relationships in cystic fibrosis. *Medical Clinics of North America*, *84*(3), 597-607.

[60] Hamosh, A., Grade, K., Coutelle, C. and Reis, A. (1993). Correlation between genotype and phenotype in patients with cystic fibrosis. *New England Journal of Medicine*, *329*(18), 1308-1313.

[61] Rowntree, R. K. and Harris, A. (2003). The phenotypic consequences of CFTR mutations. *Annals of Human Genetics*, *67*(5), 471-485.

[62] Wilschanski, M., Yahav, Y., Yaacov, Y., Blau, H., Bentur, L., Rivlin, J., et al. (2003). Gentamicin-induced correction of CFTR function in patients with cystic fibrosis and CFTR stop mutations. *New England Journal of Medicine*, *349*(15), 1433-1441.

[63] Wahab, A. A., Janahi, I. A. and Marafia, M. M. (2004). Pseudo-Bartter's syndrome in an Egyptian infant with cystic fibrosis mutation N1303K. *Journal of Tropical Pediatrics*, *50*(4), 242-244.

[64] Wang, Y., Bartlett, M. C., Loo, T. W. and Clarke, D. M. (2006). Specific rescue of cystic fibrosis transmembrane conductance regulator processing mutants using pharmacological chaperones. *Molecular Pharmacology*, *70*(1), 297-302.

[65] Howell, L. D., Borchardt, R. and Cohn, J. A. (2000). ATP hydrolysis by a CFTR domain: pharmacology and effects of G551D mutation. *Biochemical and Biophysical Research Communications*, *271*(2), 518-525.

[66] Choi, J. Y., Muallem, D., Kiselyov, K., Lee, M. G., Thomas, P. J. and Muallem, S. (2001). Aberrant CFTR-dependent HCO_3^- transport in mutations associated with cystic fibrosis. *Nature*, *410*(6824), 94-97.

[67] Molinski, S. V., Gonska, T., Huan, L. J., Baskin, B., Janahi, I. A., Ray, P. N. and Bear, C. E. (2014). Genetic, cell biological, and clinical interrogation of the CFTR mutation c. 3700 A> G (p. Ile1234Val) informs strategies for future medical intervention. *Genetics in Medicine*, *16*(8), 625-632.

[68] Moran, O. (2010). Model of the cAMP activation of chloride transport by CFTR channel and the mechanism of potentiators. *Journal of Theoretical Biology*, *262*(1), 73-79.

[69] Aznarez, I., Chan, E. M., Zielenski, J., Blencowe, B. J. and Tsui, L. C. (2003). Characterization of disease-associated mutations affecting an exonic splicing enhancer and two cryptic splice sites in exon 13 of the cystic fibrosis transmembrane conductance regulator gene. *Human Molecular Genetics*, *12*(16), 2031-2040.

[70] Zuccato, E., Buratti, E., Stuani, C., Baralle, F. E. and Pagani, F. (2004). An intronic polypyrimidine-rich element downstream of the donor site modulates cystic fibrosis transmembrane conductance regulator exon 9 alternative splicing. *Journal of Biological Chemistry*, *279*(17), 16980-16988.

[71] Zielenski, J. (2000). Genotype and phenotype in cystic fibrosis. *Respiration*, *67*(2), 117-133.

[72] Ostedgaard, L. S., Randak, C., Rokhlina, T., Karp, P., Vermeer, D., Excoffon, K. J. A. and Welsh, M. J. (2003). Effects of C-terminal deletions on cystic fibrosis transmembrane conductance regulator

function in cystic fibrosis airway epithelia. *Proceedings of the National Academy of Sciences*, *100*(4), 1937-1942.

[73] Quinton, P. M. (2007). Cystic fibrosis: lessons from the sweat gland. *Physiology*, *22*(3), 212-22

[74] Morgan, R. M., Patterson, M. J. and Nimmo, M. A. (2004). Acute effects of dehydration on sweat composition in men during prolonged exercise in the heat. *Acta Physiologica Scandinavica*, *182*(1), 37-43.

[75] Brown, M. B., Haack, K. K., Pollack, B. P., Millard-Stafford, M. and McCarty, N. A. (2011). Low abundance of sweat duct Cl^- channel CFTR in both healthy and cystic fibrosis athletes with exceptionally salty sweat during exercise. *American Journal of Physiology-Regulatory, Integrative and Comparative Physiology*, *300*(3), R605-R615.

[76] Quinton, P. M. (1999). Physiological basis of cystic fibrosis: a historical perspective. *Physiological Reviews*, *79*(1), S3-S22.

[77] Hammond, K. B., Turcios, N. L. and Gibson, L. E. (1994). Clinical evaluation of the macroduct sweat collection system and conductivity analyzer in the diagnosis of cystic fibrosis. *The Journal of Pediatrics*, *124*(2), 255-260.

[78] Rosenstein, B. J. and Cutting, G. R. (1998). The diagnosis of cystic fibrosis: a consensus statement. *The Journal of Pediatrics*, *132*(4), 589-595.

[79] Stern, R. C. (1997). The diagnosis of cystic fibrosis. *New England Journal of Medicine*, *336*(7), 487-491.

[80] Matsui, H., Grubb, B. R., Tarran, R., Randell, S. H., Gatzy, J. T., Davis, C. W. and Boucher, R. C. (1998). Evidence for periciliary liquid layer depletion, not abnormal ion composition, in the pathogenesis of cystic fibrosis airways disease. *Cell*, *95*(7), 1005-1015.

[81] Widdicombe, J. H. and Widdicombe, J. G. (1995). Regulation of human airway surface liquid. *Respiration Physiology*, *99*(1), 3-12.

[82] Boucher, R. C. (2007). Airway surface dehydration in cystic fibrosis: pathogenesis and therapy. *Annual Review of Medicine*, *58*, 157-170.

[83] Boucher, R. C. (2004). New concepts of the pathogenesis of cystic fibrosis lung disease. *European Respiratory Journal*, *23*(1), 146-158.

[84] Konstan, M. W. and Berger, M. (1997). Current understanding of the inflammatory process in cystic fibrosis: Onset and etiology. *Pediatric Pulmonology*, *24*, 137-142.

[85] Koch, C. (2002). Early infection and progression of cystic fibrosis lung disease. *Pediatric Pulmonology*, *34*(3), 232-236.

[86] Costerton, J. W. (2001). Cystic fibrosis pathogenesis and the role of biofilms in persistent infection. *Trends in Microbiology*, *9*(2), 50-52.

[87] Li, Z., Kosorok, M. R., Farrell, P. M., Laxova, A., West, S. E., Green, C. G., et al. (2005). Longitudinal development of mucoid *Pseudomonas aeruginosa* infection and lung disease progression in children with cystic fibrosis. *JAMA, 293*(5), 581-588.

[88] Lai, H. J., Cheng, Y., Cho, H., Kosorok, M. R. and Farrell, P. M. (2004). Association between initial disease presentation, lung disease outcomes, and survival in patients with cystic fibrosis. *American Journal of Epidemiology*, *159*(6), 537-546.

[89] Wilschanski, M., Dupuis, A., Ellis, L., Jarvi, K., Zielenski, J., Tullis, E., et al. (2006). Mutations in the cystic fibrosis transmembrane regulator gene and in vivo transepithelial potentials. *American Journal of Respiratory and Critical Care Medicine*, *174*(7), 787-794.

[90] Standaert, T. A., Boitano, L., Emerson, J., Milgram, L. J., Konstan, M. W., Hunter, J., et al. (2004). Standardized procedure for measurement of nasal potential difference: an outcome measure in multicenter cystic fibrosis clinical trials. *Pediatric Pulmonology*, *37*(5), 385-392.

[91] Wilschanski, M., Famini, H., Strauss-Liviatan, N., Rivlin, J., Blau, H., Bibi, H., et al. (2001). Nasal potential difference measurements in patients with atypical cystic fibrosis. *European Respiratory Journal*, *17*(6), 1208-1215.

[92] Farrell, P. M., Rosenstein, B. J., White, T. B., Accurso, F. J., Castellani, C., Cutting, G. R., et al. (2008). Guidelines for diagnosis of cystic fibrosis in newborns through older adults: Cystic Fibrosis Foundation consensus report. *The Journal of Pediatrics*, *153*(2), S4-S14.

[93] Gysin, C., Alothman, G. A. and Papsin, B. C. (2000). Sinonasal disease in cystic fibrosis: clinical characteristics, diagnosis, and management. *Pediatric Pulmonology*, *30*(6), 481-489.

[94] Hadfield, P. J., Rowe-Jones, J. M. and Mackay, I. S. (2000). The prevalence of nasal polyps in adults with cystic fibrosis. *Clinical Otolaryngology and Allied Sciences*, *25*(1), 19-22.

[95] Wang, X., Moylan, B., Leopold, D. A., Kim, J., Rubenstein, R. C., Togias, A., et al. (2000). Mutation in the gene responsible for cystic

fibrosis and predisposition to chronic rhinosinusitis in the general population. *JAMA*, *284*(14), 1814-1819.
[96] Woodworth, B. A., Ahn, C., Flume, P. A. and Schlosser, R. J. (2007). The delta F508 mutation in cystic fibrosis and impact on sinus development. *American Journal of Rhinology*, *21*(1), 122-127.
[97] Durno, C., Corey, M., Zielenski, J., Tullis, E., Tsui, L. C. and Durie, P. (2002). Genotype and phenotype correlations in patients with cystic fibrosis and pancreatitis. *Gastroenterology*, *123*(6), 1857-1864.
[98] Sheppard, M. N. and Nicholson, A. G. (2002). The pathology of cystic fibrosis. *Current Diagnostic Pathology*, *8*(1), 50-59.
[99] Moran, A., Dunitz, J., Nathan, B., Saeed, A., Holme, B. and Thomas, W. (2009). Cystic fibrosis–related diabetes: current trends in prevalence, incidence, and mortality. *Diabetes Care*, *32*(9), 1626-1631.
[100] Rolon, M. A., Benali, K., Munck, A., Navarro, J., Clement, A., Tubiana-Rufi, N., et al. (2001). Cystic fibrosis-related diabetes mellitus: clinical impact of prediabetes and effects of insulin therapy. *Acta Paediatrica*, *90*(8), 860-867.
[101] Wouthuyzen-Bakker, M., Bodewes, F. A. and Verkade, H. J. (2011). Persistent fat malabsorption in cystic fibrosis; lessons from patients and mice. *Journal of Cystic Fibrosis*, *10*(3), 150-158.
[102] Munck, A., Gérardin, M., Alberti, C., Ajzenman, C., Lebourgeois, M., Aigrain, Y. and Navarro, J. (2006). Clinical outcome of cystic fibrosis presenting with or without meconium ileus: a matched cohort study. *Journal of Pediatric Surgery*, *41*(9), 1556-1560.
[103] van der Doef, H. P., Kokke, F. T., van der Ent, C. K. and Houwen, R. H. (2011). Intestinal obstruction syndromes in cystic fibrosis: meconium ileus, distal intestinal obstruction syndrome, and constipation. *Current Gastroenterology Reports*, *13*(3), 265-270.
[104] Houwen, R. H., van der Doef, H. P., Sermet, I., Munck, A., Hauser, B., Walkowiak, J., et al. (2010). Defining DIOS and constipation in cystic fibrosis with a multicentre study on the incidence, characteristics, and treatment of DIOS. *Journal of Pediatric Gastroenterology and Nutrition*, *50*(1), 38-42.
[105] Colombo, C., Russo, M. C., Zazzeron, L. and Romano, G. (2006). Liver disease in cystic fibrosis. *Journal of Pediatric Gastroenterology and Nutrition*, *43*(1), S49-S55.

[106] Moyer, K. and Balistreri, W. (2009). Hepatobiliary disease in patients with cystic fibrosis. *Current Opinion in Gastroenterology*, *25*(3), 272-278.

[107] Bartlett, J. R., Friedman, K. J., Ling, S. C., Pace, R. G., Bell, S. C., Bourke, B., et al. (2009). Genetic modifiers of liver disease in cystic fibrosis. *JAMA*, *302*(10), 1076-1083.

[108] Chaudry, G., Navarro, O. M., Levine, D. S. and Oudjhane, K. (2006). Abdominal manifestations of cystic fibrosis in children. *Pediatric Radiology*, *36*(3), 233-240.

[109] Bezerra, J. A. (2005). Potential etiologies of biliary atresia. *Pediatric Transplantation*, *9*(5), 646-651.

[110] Xu, W. M., Shi, Q. X., Chen, W. Y., Zhou, C. X., Ni, Y., Rowlands, D. K., et al. (2007). Cystic fibrosis transmembrane conductance regulator is vital to sperm fertilizing capacity and male fertility. *Proceedings of the National Academy of Sciences*, *104*(23), 9816-9821.

[111] Escobar, M. A., Grosfeld, J. L., Burdick, J. J., Powell, R. L., Jay, C. L., Wait, A. D., et al. (2005). Surgical considerations in cystic fibrosis: a 32-year evaluation of outcomes. *Surgery*, *138*(4), 560-572.

[112] Yu, J., Chen, Z., Ni, Y. and Li, Z. (2012). CFTR mutations in men with congenital bilateral absence of the vas deferens (CBAVD): a systemic review and meta-analysis. *Human Reproduction*, *27*(1), 25-35.

[113] Hodges, C. A., Palmert, M. R. and Drumm, M. L. (2008). Infertility in females with cystic fibrosis is multifactorial: evidence from mouse models. *Endocrinology*, *149*(6), 2790-2797.

[114] Aris, R. M., Merkel, P. A., Bachrach, L. K., Borowitz, D. S., Boyle, M. P., Elkin, S. L., et al. (2005). Guide to bone health and disease in cystic fibrosis. *The Journal of Clinical Endocrinology and Metabolism*, *90*(3), 1888-1896.

[115] Paccou, J., Zeboulon, N., Combescure, C., Gossec, L. and Cortet, B. (2010). The prevalence of osteoporosis, osteopenia, and fractures among adults with cystic fibrosis: a systematic literature review with meta-analysis. *Calcified Tissue International*, *86*(1), 1-7.

[116] Rovner, A. J., Stallings, V. A., Schall, J. I., Leonard, M. B. and Zemel, B. S. (2007). Vitamin D insufficiency in children, adolescents, and young adults with cystic fibrosis despite routine oral supplementation. *The American Journal of Clinical Nutrition*, *86*(6), 1694-1699.

[117] Cutting, G. R. (2010). Modifier genes in Mendelian disorders: the example of cystic fibrosis. *Annals of the New York Academy of Sciences, 1214*(1), 57-69.

[118] Darmstadt, G. L., Schmidt, C. P., Wechsler, D. S., Tunnessen, W. W. and Rosenstein, B. J. (1992). Dermatitis as a presenting sign of cystic fibrosis. *Archives of Dermatology, 128*(10), 1358-1364.

[119] Zahraldin, K., Janahi, I. A., Ben-Omran, T., Alsulaiman, R., Hamad, B. and Imam, A. (2015). Two Qatari siblings with cystic fibrosis and apparent mineralocorticoid excess. *Annals of Thoracic Medicine, 10*(1), 69.

[120] Wilfond, B. S., Farrell, P. M., Laxova, A. and Mischler, E. (1994). Severe hemolytic anemia associated with vitamin E deficiency in infants with cystic fibrosis: Implications for neonatal screening. *Clinical pediatrics, 33*(1), 2-7.

[121] Kerem, E., Conway, S., Elborn, S. and Heijerman, H. for the Consensus Committee. (2005). Standards of care for patients with cystic fibrosis: a European consensus. *Journal of Cystic Fibrosis, 4*(1), 7-26.

[122] Boyle, M. P. (2007). Adult cystic fibrosis. *JAMA, 298*(15), 1787-1793.

[123] Stallings, V. A., Stark, L. J., Robinson, K. A., Feranchak, A. P., Quinton, H., Clinical Practice Guidelines on Growth and Nutrition Subcommittee; Ad Hoc Working Group. (2008). Evidence-based practice recommendations for nutrition-related management of children and adults with cystic fibrosis and pancreatic insufficiency: results of a systematic review. *Journal of the American Dietetic Association, 108*(5), 832-839.

[124] Langfelder-Schwind, E., Karczeski, B., Strecker, M. N., Redman, J., Sugarman, E. A., Zaleski, C., et al. (2014). Molecular testing for cystic fibrosis carrier status practice guidelines: recommendations of the National Society of Genetic Counselors. *Journal of Genetic Counseling, 23*(1), 5-15.

[125] Egan, M. E., Green, D. M. and Voynow, J. A. (2016). Cystic Fibrosis. In: Kliegman, R. M., Stanton, B., St. Geme, J. and Schor, N. (Eds.), *Nelson Textbook of Pediatrics* (20th edition, pp. 2098-2113). Amsterdam, Netherlands: Elsevier, Inc.

[126] Dequeker, E., Stuhrmann, M., Morris, M. A., Casals, T., Castellani, C., Claustres, M., et al. (2009). Best practice guidelines for molecular genetic diagnosis of cystic fibrosis and CFTR-related disorders–updated

European recommendations. *European Journal of Human Genetics*, *17*(1), 51-65.

[127] Boyle, M. P. (2003). Nonclassic cystic fibrosis and CFTR-related diseases. *Current Opinion in Pulmonary Medicine*, *9*(6), 498-503.

[128] Gibson, R. L., Burns, J. L. and Ramsey, B. W. (2003). Pathophysiology and management of pulmonary infections in cystic fibrosis. *American Journal of Respiratory and Critical Care Medicine*, *168*(8), 918-951.

[129] Sawicki, G. S., Sellers, D. E. and Robinson, W. M. (2009). High treatment burden in adults with cystic fibrosis: challenges to disease self-management. *Journal of Cystic Fibrosis*, *8*(2), 91-96.

[130] Wheatley, C. M., Wilkins, B. W. and Snyder, E. M. (2011). Exercise is medicine in cystic fibrosis. *Exercise and Sport Sciences Reviews*, *39*(3), 155-160.

[131] Flume, P. A., Mogayzel Jr, P. J., Robinson, K. A., Goss, C. H., Rosenblatt, R. L., Kuhn, R. J. and Marshall, B. C. (2009). Cystic fibrosis pulmonary guidelines: treatment of pulmonary exacerbations. *American Journal of Respiratory and Critical Care Medicine*, *180*(9), 802-808.

[132] Nielsen, K. G., Pressler, T., Klug, B., Koch, C. and Bisgaard, H. (2004). Serial lung function and responsiveness in cystic fibrosis during early childhood. *American Journal of Respiratory and Critical Care Medicine*, *169*(11), 1209-1216.

[133] Flume, P. A., Robinson, K. A., O'Sullivan, B. P., Finder, J. D., Vender, R. L., Willey-Courand, D. B., et al. (2009). Cystic fibrosis pulmonary guidelines: airway clearance therapies. *Respiratory Care*, *54*(4), 522-537.

[134] Hess, D. R. (2007). Airway clearance: physiology, pharmacology, techniques, and practice. *Respiratory Care*, *52*(10), 1392-1396.

[135] Quan, J. M., Tiddens, H. A., Sy, J. P., McKenzie, S. G., Montgomery, M. D., Robinson, P. J., et al. (2001). A two-year randomized, placebo-controlled trial of dornase alfa in young patients with cystic fibrosis with mild lung function abnormalities. *The Journal of Pediatrics*, *139*(6), 813-820.

[136] Donaldson, S. H., Bennett, W. D., Zeman, K. L., Knowles, M. R., Tarran, R. and Boucher, R. C. (2006). Mucus clearance and lung function in cystic fibrosis with hypertonic saline. *New England Journal of Medicine*, *354*(3), 241-250.

[137] Balfour-Lynn, I. M. and Welch, K. (2014). Inhaled corticosteroids for cystic fibrosis. *Cochrane Database of Systematic Reviews, 10*, CD001915.

[138] Flume, P. A., O'Sullivan, B. P., Robinson, K. A., Goss, C. H., Mogayzel Jr, P. J., Willey-Courand, D. B., et al. (2007). Cystic fibrosis pulmonary guidelines: chronic medications for maintenance of lung health. *American Journal of Respiratory and Critical Care Medicine*, *176*(10), 957-969.

[139] Konstan, M. W., Schluchter, M. D., Xue, W. and Davis, P. B. (2007). Clinical use of ibuprofen is associated with slower FEV1 decline in children with cystic fibrosis. *American Journal of Respiratory and Critical Care Medicine*, *176*(11), 1084-1089.

[140] Cai, Y., Chai, D., Wang, R., Bai, N., Liang, B. B. and Liu, Y. (2011). Effectiveness and safety of macrolides in cystic fibrosis patients: a meta-analysis and systematic review. *Journal of Antimicrobial Chemotherapy*, *66*(5), 968-978.

[141] Döring, G. and Hoiby, N. for the Consensus Study Group. (2004). Early intervention and prevention of lung disease in cystic fibrosis: a European consensus. *Journal of Cystic Fibrosis*, *3*(2), 67-91.

[142] Janahi, I. A., Abdulwahab, A., Sittana, S. E. and Bush, A. (2005). Rapidly progressive lung disease in a patient with cystic fibrosis on long-term azithromycin: possible role of mycoplasma infection. *Journal of Cystic Fibrosis*, *4*(1), 71-73.

[143] Rosenfeld, M., Emerson, J., Williams-Warren, J., Pepe, M., Smith, A., Montgomery, A. B. and Ramsey, B. (2001). Defining a pulmonary exacerbation in cystic fibrosis. *The Journal of Pediatrics*, *139*(3), 359-365.

[144] Ratjen, F. (2001). Changes in strategies for optimal antibacterial therapy in cystic fibrosis. *International Journal of Antimicrobial Agents*, *17*(2), 93-96.

[145] Flume, P. A., Mogayzel Jr, P. J., Robinson, K. A., Goss, C. H., Rosenblatt, R. L., Kuhn, R. J. and Marshall, B. C. (2009). Cystic fibrosis pulmonary guidelines: treatment of pulmonary exacerbations. *American Journal of Respiratory and Critical Care Medicine*, *180*(9), 802-808.

[146] Stevens, D. A., Moss, R. B., Kurup, V. P., Knutsen, A. P., Greenberger, P., Judson, M. A., et al. (2003). Allergic bronchopulmonary aspergillosis

in cystic fibrosis—state of the art: Cystic Fibrosis Foundation Consensus Conference. *Clinical Infectious Diseases*, *37*(Supplement 3), S225-S264.

[147] Olivier, K. N., Weber, D. J., Lee, J. H., Handler, A., Tudor, G., Molina, P. L., et al. (2003). Nontuberculous mycobacteria: II: nested-cohort study of impact on cystic fibrosis lung disease. *American Journal of Respiratory and Critical Care Medicine*, *167*(6), 835-840.

[148] Wahab, A. A., Janahi, I. A., Marafia, M. M. and El-Shafie, S. (2004). Microbiological identification in cystic fibrosis patients with CFTR I1234V mutation. *Journal of Tropical Pediatrics*, *50*(4), 229-233.

[149] Conway, S. P., Brownlee, K. G., Denton, M. and Peckham, D. G. (2003). Antibiotic treatment of multidrug-resistant organisms in cystic fibrosis. *American Journal of Respiratory Medicine*, *2*(4), 321-332.

[150] Valenza, G., Tappe, D., Turnwald, D., Frosch, M., König, C., Hebestreit, H. and Abele-Horn, M. (2008). Prevalence and antimicrobial susceptibility of microorganisms isolated from sputa of patients with cystic fibrosis. *Journal of Cystic Fibrosis*, *7*(2), 123-127.

[151] Besier, S., Smaczny, C., von Mallinckrodt, C., Krahl, A., Ackermann, H., Brade, V. and Wichelhaus, T. A. (2007). Prevalence and clinical significance of *Staphylococcus aureus* small-colony variants in cystic fibrosis lung disease. *Journal of Clinical Microbiology*, *45*(1), 168-172.

[152] Dasenbrook, E. C., Merlo, C. A., Diener-West, M., Lechtzin, N. and Boyle, M. P. (2008). Persistent methicillin-resistant *Staphylococcus aureus* and rate of FEV1 decline in cystic fibrosis. *American Journal of Respiratory and Critical Care Medicine*, *178*(8), 814-821.

[153] Li, Z., Kosorok, M. R., Farrell, P. M., Laxova, A., West, S. E., Green, C. G., et al. (2005). Longitudinal development of mucoid *Pseudomonas aeruginosa* infection and lung disease progression in children with cystic fibrosis. *JAMA*, *293*(5), 581-588.

[154] Döring, G., Conway, S. P., Heijerman, H. G. M., Hodson, M. E., Høiby, N., Smyth, A., et al. (2000). Antibiotic therapy against *Pseudomonas aeruginosa* in cystic fibrosis: a European consensus. *European Respiratory Journal*, *16*(4), 749-767.

[155] Waters, V. and Ratjen, F. (2006). Multidrug–resistant organisms in cystic fibrosis: management and infection–control issues. *Expert Review of Anti-Infective Therapy*, *4*(5), 807-819.

[156] Wahab, A. A., Janahi, I. A. and El-Shafie, S. S. (2004). *Achromobacter xylosoxidans* isolated from the sputum of a patient with cystic fibrosis

mutation I1234V with *Pseudomonas aeruginosa. Saudi Medical Journal*, *25*(6), 810-811.

[157] Aaron, S. D., Ferris, W., Henry, D. A., Speert, D. P. and MacDonald, N. E. (2000). Multiple combination bactericidal antibiotic testing for patients with cystic fibrosis infected with *Burkholderia cepacia*. *American Journal of Respiratory and Critical Care Medicine*, *161*(4), 1206-1212.

[158] Jones, A. M., Dodd, M. E., Govan, J. R. W., Barcus, V., Doherty, C. J., Morris, J. and Webb, A. K. (2004). *Burkholderia cenocepacia* and *Burkholderia multivorans*: influence on survival in cystic fibrosis. *Thorax*, *59*(11), 948-951.

[159] Young, A. C., Wilson, J. W., Kotsimbos, T. C. and Naughton, M. T. (2008). Randomised placebo controlled trial of non-invasive ventilation for hypercapnia in cystic fibrosis. *Thorax*, *63*(1), 72-77.

[160] Millis, R. M., Young, R. C. and Kulczycki, L. L. (1977). Validation of therapeutic bronchoscopic bronchial washing in cystic fibrosis. *CHEST Journal*, *71*(4), 508-513.

[161] Flume, P. A. (2003). Pneumothorax in cystic fibrosis. *CHEST Journal*, *123*(1), 217-221.

[162] Flume, P. A., Mogayzel Jr, P. J., Robinson, K. A., Rosenblatt, R. L., Quittell, L. and Marshall, B. C. (2010). Cystic fibrosis pulmonary guidelines: pulmonary complications: hemoptysis and pneumothorax. *American Journal of Respiratory and Critical Care Medicine*, *182*(3), 298-306.

[163] Orens, J. B., Estenne, M., Arcasoy, S., Conte, J. V., Corris, P., Egan, J. J., et al. (2006). International guidelines for the selection of lung transplant candidates: 2006 update—a consensus report from the Pulmonary Scientific Council of the International Society for Heart and Lung Transplantation. *The Journal of Heart and Lung Transplantation*, *25*(7), 745-755.

[164] Borowitz, D., Baker, R. D. and Stallings, V. (2002). Consensus report on nutrition for pediatric patients with cystic fibrosis. *Journal of Pediatric Gastroenterology and Nutrition*, *35*(3), 246-259.

[165] Blondeau, K., Dupont, L. J., Mertens, V., Verleden, G., Malfroot, A., Vandenplas, Y., et al. (2008). Gastro-oesophageal reflux and aspiration of gastric contents in adult patients with cystic fibrosis. *Gut*, *57*(8), 1049-1055.

[166] Colombo, C., Ellemunter, H., Houwen, R., Munck, A., Taylor, C. and Wilschanski, M. (2011). Guidelines for the diagnosis and management of distal intestinal obstruction syndrome in cystic fibrosis patients. *Journal of Cystic Fibrosis*, *10*, S24-S28.

[167] Ode, K. L., Frohnert, B., Laguna, T., Phillips, J., Holme, B., Regelmann, W., et al. (2010). Oral glucose tolerance testing in children with cystic fibrosis. *Pediatric Diabetes*, *11*(7), 487-492.

[168] Tofé, S., Moreno, J. C., Máiz, L., Alonso, M., Escobar, H. and Barrio, R. (2005). Insulin-secretion abnormalities and clinical deterioration related to impaired glucose tolerance in cystic fibrosis. *European Journal of Endocrinology*, *152*(2), 241-247.

[169] Moran, A., Brunzell, C., Cohen, R. C., Katz, M., Marshall, B. C., Onady, G., et al. (2010). Clinical Care Guidelines for Cystic Fibrosis–Related Diabetes: A position statement of the American Diabetes Association and a clinical practice guideline of the Cystic Fibrosis Foundation, endorsed by the Pediatric Endocrine Society. *Diabetes Care*, *33*(12), 2697-2708.

[170] Sermet-Gaudelus, I., Bianchi, M. L., Garabédian, M., Aris, R. M., Morton, A., Hardin, D. S., et al. (2011). European cystic fibrosis bone mineralisation guidelines. *Journal of Cystic Fibrosis*, *10*, S16-S23.

[171] Beker, L. T., Russek-Cohen, E. and Fink, R. J. (2001). Stature as a prognostic factor in cystic fibrosis survival. *Journal of the American Dietetic Association*, *101*(4), 438-442.

[172] Hardin, D. S., Adams-Huet, B., Brown, D., Chatfield, B., Dyson, M., Ferkol, T., et al. (2006). Growth hormone treatment improves growth and clinical status in prepubertal children with cystic fibrosis: results of a multicenter randomized controlled trial. *The Journal of Clinical Endocrinology and Metabolism*, *91*(12), 4925-4929.

[173] Khalil, H. S. and Nunez, D. A. (2006). Functional endoscopic sinus surgery for chronic rhinosinusitis. *Cochrane Database of Systematic Reviews*, *3*, CD004458.

[174] Fustik, S., Pop-Jordanova, N., Slaveska, N., Koceva, S. and Efremov, G. (2002). Metabolic alkalosis with hypoelectrolytemia in infants with cystic fibrosis. *Pediatrics International*, *44*(3), 289-292.

[175] Popli, K. and Stewart, J. (2007). Infertility and its management in men with cystic fibrosis: review of literature and clinical practices in the UK. *Human Fertility*, *10*(4), 217-221.

[176] Quittner, A. L., Barker, D. H., Snell, C., Grimley, M. E., Marciel, K. and Cruz, I. (2008). Prevalence and impact of depression in cystic fibrosis. *Current Opinion in Pulmonary Medicine*, *14*(6), 582-588.

[177] Sands, D., Repetto, T., Dupont, L. J., Korzeniewska-Eksterowicz, A., Catastini, P. and Madge, S. (2011). End of life care for patients with cystic fibrosis. *Journal of Cystic Fibrosis*, *10*, S37-S44.

[178] Clancy, J. P. and Jain, M. (2012). Personalized medicine in cystic fibrosis: dawning of a new era. *American Journal of Respiratory and Critical Care Medicine*, *186*(7), 593-597.

[179] Lindee, S. and Mueller, R. (2011). Is cystic fibrosis genetic medicine's canary? *Perspectives in Biology and Medicine*, *54*(3), 316-331.

[180] Selkirk, S. M. (2004). Gene therapy in clinical medicine. *Postgraduate Medical Journal*, *80*(948), 560-570.

[181] Dobson, J. (2006). Gene therapy progress and prospects: magnetic nanoparticle-based gene delivery. *Gene Therapy*, *13*(4), 283-287.

[182] Ferrari, S., Geddes, D. M. and Alton, E. W. (2002). Barriers to and new approaches for gene therapy and gene delivery in cystic fibrosis. *Advanced Drug Delivery Reviews*, *54*(11), 1373-1393.

[183] Bilton, D. (2015). A new chapter in therapy for cystic fibrosis. *The Lancet Respiratory Medicine*, *3*(7), e20.

[184] Pedemonte, N., Lukacs, G. L., Du, K., Caci, E., Zegarra-Moran, O., Galietta, L. J. and Verkman, A. S. (2005). Small-molecule correctors of defective ΔF508-CFTR cellular processing identified by high-throughput screening. *The Journal of Clinical Investigation*, *115*(9), 2564-2571.

[185] Ramsey, B. W., Davies, J., McElvaney, N. G., Tullis, E., Bell, S. C., Dřevínek, P., et al. (2011). A CFTR potentiator in patients with cystic fibrosis and the G551D mutation. *New England Journal of Medicine*, *365*(18), 1663-1672.

[186] Clancy, J. P., Rowe, S. M., Accurso, F. J., Aitken, M. L., Amin, R. S., Ashlock, M. A., et al. (2012). Results of a phase IIa study of VX-809, an investigational CFTR corrector compound, in subjects with cystic fibrosis homozygous for the F508del-CFTR mutation. *Thorax*, *67*(1), 12-18.

[187] Wainwright, C. E., Elborn, J. S., Ramsey, B. W., Marigowda, G., Huang, X., Cipolli, M., et al. (2015). Lumacaftor–ivacaftor in patients

with cystic fibrosis homozygous for Phe508del CFTR. *New England Journal of Medicine*, *373*(3), 220-231.

[188] Hutt, D. M., Herman, D., Rodrigues, A. P., Noel, S., Pilewski, J. M., Matteson, J., et al. (2010). Reduced histone deacetylase 7 activity restores function to misfolded CFTR in cystic fibrosis. *Nature Chemical Biology*, *6*(1), 25-33.

[189] Davidson, B. L. and McCray, P. B. (2011). Current prospects for RNA interference-based therapies. *Nature Reviews Genetics*, *12*(5), 329-340.

[190] Sazani, P. and Kole, R. (2003). Therapeutic potential of antisense oligonucleotides as modulators of alternative splicing. *The Journal of Clinical Investigation*, *112*(4), 481-486.

[191] Sermet-Gaudelus, I., Boeck, K. D., Casimir, G. J., Vermeulen, F., Leal, T., Mogenet, A., et al. (2010). Ataluren (PTC124) induces cystic fibrosis transmembrane conductance regulator protein expression and activity in children with nonsense mutation cystic fibrosis. *American Journal of Respiratory and Critical Care Medicine*, *182*(10), 1262-1272.

[192] Rehman, A., Baloch, N. U., Janahi, I. A. (2015) Lumacaftor-ivacaftor in patients with cystic fibrosis homozygous for Phe508del CFTR. *New England Journal of Medicine*, *373*(18), 1783.

[193] Rehman, A., Awais, M., Baloch, N. U. (2016) Precision medicine and low- to middle-income countries. *JAMA Oncology*, *2*(3), 293-294.

[194] Tiddens, H. A., Puderbach, M., Venegas, J. G., Ratjen, F., Donaldson, S. H., Davis, S. D., et al. (2015). Novel outcome measures for clinical trials in cystic fibrosis. *Pediatric Pulmonology*, *50*(3), 302-315.

[195] Milla, C. E. and Warwick, W. J. (1998). Risk of death in cystic fibrosis patients with severely compromised lung function. *CHEST Journal*, *113*(5), 1230-1234.

[196] Tiddens, H. A. (2002). Detecting early structural lung damage in cystic fibrosis. *Pediatric Pulmonology*, *34*(3), 228-231.

[197] Lum, S., Stocks, J., Castile, R. and Davis, S. (2005). ATS/ERS statement: raised volume forced expirations in infants: guidelines for current practice. *American Journal of Respiratory and Critical Care Medicine*, *172*(11), 1463.

[198] Davis, S. D., Rosenfeld, M., Kerby, G. S., Brumback, L., Kloster, M. H., Acton, J. D., et al. (2010). Multicenter evaluation of infant lung function tests as cystic fibrosis clinical trial endpoints. *American Journal of Respiratory and Critical Care Medicine*, *182*(11), 1387-1397.

[199] Aurora, P., Bush, A., Gustafsson, P., Oliver, C., Wallis, C., Price, J., et al. (2005). Multiple-breath washout as a marker of lung disease in preschool children with cystic fibrosis. *American Journal of Respiratory and Critical Care Medicine*, *171*(3), 249-256.

[200] Aurora, P., Gustafsson, P., Bush, A., Lindblad, A., Oliver, C., Wallis, C. E. and Stocks, J. (2004). Multiple breath inert gas washout as a measure of ventilation distribution in children with cystic fibrosis. *Thorax*, *59*(12), 1068-1073.

[201] Horsley, A. R., Gustafsson, P. M., Macleod, K. A., Saunders, C., Greening, A. P., Porteous, D. J., et al. (2008). Lung clearance index is a sensitive, repeatable and practical measure of airways disease in adults with cystic fibrosis. *Thorax*, *63*(2), 135-140.

[202] Gustafsson, P. M., de Jong, P. A., Tiddens, H. A. and Lindblad, A. (2008). Multiple-breath inert gas washout and spirometry versus structural lung disease in cystic fibrosis. *Thorax*, *63*(2), 129-134.

[203] Lum, S., Gustafsson, P., Ljungberg, H., Hülskamp, G., Bush, A., Carr, S. B., et al. (2007). Early detection of cystic fibrosis lung disease: multiple-breath washout versus raised volume tests. *Thorax*, *62*(4), 341-347.

[204] Mott, L. S., Park, J., Murray, C. P., Gangell, C. L., de Klerk, N. H., Robinson, P. J., et al. (2011). Progression of early structural lung disease in young children with cystic fibrosis assessed using CT. *Thorax*, *67*(5), 509-516.

[205] Bhat, V., Wahab, A. A., Garg, K. C., Janahi, I. and Singh, R. (2015). HRCT in cystic fibrosis in patients with CFTR I1234V mutation: Assessment of scoring systems with low dose technique using multidetector system and correlation with pulmonary function tests. *The Indian Journal of Radiology and Imaging*, *25*(1), 44-51.

[206] Brody, A. S., Kosorok, M. R., Li, Z., Broderick, L. S., Foster, J. L., Laxova, A., et al. (2006). Reproducibility of a scoring system for computed tomography scanning in cystic fibrosis. *Journal of Thoracic Imaging*, *21*(1), 14-21.

[207] Mayo, J. R., Aldrich, J. and Muller, N. L. (2003). Radiation exposure at chest CT: a statement of the Fleischner Society. *Radiology*, *228*(1), 15-21.

[208] Failo, R., Wielopolski, P. A., Tiddens, H. A., Hop, W. C., Pozzi Mucelli, R. and Lequin, M. H. (2009). Lung morphology assessment using MRI:

A robust ultra-short TR/TE 2D steady state free precession sequence used in cystic fibrosis patients. *Magnetic Resonance in Medicine*, *61*(2), 299-306.

[209] Puderbach, M., Eichinger, M., Haeselbarth, J., Ley, S., Kopp-Schneider, A., Tuengerthal, S., et al. (2007). Assessment of morphological MRI for pulmonary changes in cystic fibrosis (CF) patients: comparison to thin-section CT and chest x-ray. *Investigative Radiology*, *42*(10), 715-724.

[210] Klein, M., Cohen-Cymberknoh, M., Armoni, S., Shoseyov, D., Chisin, R., Orevi, M., et al. (2009). 18F-fluorodeoxyglucose-PET/CT imaging of lungs in patients with cystic fibrosis. *CHEST Journal*, *136*(5), 1220-1228.

[211] Mayer-Hamblett, N., Aitken, M. L., Accurso, F. J., Kronmal, R. A., Konstan, M. W., Burns, J. L., et al. (2007). Association between pulmonary function and sputum biomarkers in cystic fibrosis. *American Journal of Respiratory and Critical Care Medicine*, *175*(8), 822-828.

[212] Sagel, S. D., Chmiel, J. F. and Konstan, M. W. (2007). Sputum biomarkers of inflammation in cystic fibrosis lung disease. *Proceedings of the American Thoracic Society*, *4*(4), 406-417.

[213] Shoki, A. H., Mayer-Hamblett, N., Wilcox, P. G., Sin, D. D. and Quon, B. S. (2013). Systematic review of blood biomarkers in cystic fibrosis pulmonary exacerbations. *CHEST Journal*, *144*(5), 1659-1670.

[214] Levy, H., Kalish, L. A., Huntington, I., Weller, N., Gerard, C., Silverman, E. K., et al. (2007). Inflammatory markers of lung disease in adult patients with cystic fibrosis. *Pediatric Pulmonology*, *42*(3), 256-262.

[215] Koller, D. Y., Götz, M., Wojnarowski, C. and Eichler, I. (1996). Relationship between disease severity and inflammatory markers in cystic fibrosis. *Archives of Disease in Childhood*, *75*(6), 498-501.

[216] Davies, J. C., Davies, M., McShane, D., Smith, S., Chadwick, S., Jaffe, A., et al. (2005). Potential difference measurements in the lower airway of children with and without cystic fibrosis. *American Journal of Respiratory and Critical Care Medicine*, *171*(9), 1015-1019.

[217] Derichs, N., Sanz, J., Von Kanel, T., Stolpe, C., Zapf, A., Tümmler, B., et al. (2010). Intestinal current measurement for diagnostic classification of patients with questionable cystic fibrosis: validation and reference data. *Thorax*, *65*(7), 594-599.

[218] Al-Mendalawi, M. D., Abdul-Wahab, A., Janahi, I. A. and Abdel-Rahman, M. O. (2010). Sweat chloride concentration in cystic fibrosis patients with cystic fibrosis trans-membrane conductance regulator I1234V mutation. *Saudi Medical Journal*, *31*(3), 339-340.

[219] Durmowicz, A. G., Witzmann, K. A., Rosebraugh, C. J. and Chowdhury, B. A. (2013). Change in sweat chloride as a clinical end point in cystic fibrosis clinical trials: the ivacaftor experience. *CHEST Journal*, *143*(1), 14-18.

[220] Sontag, M. K., Hammond, K. B., Zielenski, J., Wagener, J. S. and Accurso, F. J. (2005). Two-tiered immunoreactive trypsinogen-based newborn screening for cystic fibrosis in Colorado: screening efficacy and diagnostic outcomes. *The Journal of Pediatrics*, *147*(3), S83-S88.

[221] Grosse, S. D., Rosenfeld, M., Devine, O. J., Lai, H. J. and Farrell, P. M. (2006). Potential impact of newborn screening for cystic fibrosis on child survival: a systematic review and analysis. *The Journal of Pediatrics*, *149*(3), 362-366.

[222] McKone, E. F., Goss, C. H. and Aitken, M. L. (2006). CFTR genotype as a predictor of prognosis in cystic fibrosis. *CHEST Journal*, *130*(5), 1441-1447.

[223] Davis, P. B., Schluchter, M. D. and Konstan, M. W. (2004). Relation of sweat chloride concentration to severity of lung disease in cystic fibrosis. *Pediatric Pulmonology*, *38*(3), 204-209.

[224] Emerson, J., Rosenfeld, M., McNamara, S., Ramsey, B. and Gibson, R. L. (2002). *Pseudomonas aeruginosa* and other predictors of mortality and morbidity in young children with cystic fibrosis. *Pediatric Pulmonology*, *34*(2), 91-100.

[225] Liou, T. G., Adler, F. R., FitzSimmons, S. C., Cahill, B. C., Hibbs, J. R. and Marshall, B. C. (2001). Predictive 5-year survivorship model of cystic fibrosis. *American Journal of Epidemiology*, *153*(4), 345-352.

[226] Emerson, J., Rosenfeld, M., McNamara, S., Ramsey, B. and Gibson, R. L. (2002). *Pseudomonas aeruginosa* and other predictors of mortality and morbidity in young children with cystic fibrosis. *Pediatric Pulmonology*, *34*(2), 91-100.

[227] Alicandro, G., Frova, L., Di Fraia, G. and Colombo, C. (2015). Cystic fibrosis mortality trend in Italy from 1970 to 2011. *Journal of Cystic Fibrosis*, *14*(2), 267-274.

[228] Mc Hugh, R., Mc Feeters, D., Boyda, D. and O'Neill, S. (2016). Coping styles in adults with cystic fibrosis: implications for emotional and social quality of life. *Psychology, Health and Medicine*, *21*(1), 102-112.

Biographical Sketch

Name: Prof. Dr. Ibrahim Ahmed M. Janahi
Affiliation: Department of Pediatrics, Hamad Medical Corporation, P.O. box 3050, Al-Rayyan Road, Doha, Qatar

Education:

1. Graduation from King Faisal University, College of Medicine and Medical Sciences, Dammam, Saudia Arabia in 1992
2. Residency in Pediatrics at University of Illinois, College of Medicine, Peoria, Illinois (USA)
3. Fellowship in Pediatric Pulmonology at Baylor College of Medicine, Houston, Texas (USA)

Address: Department of Pediatrics, Hamad Medical Corporation, P.O. box 3050, Al-Rayyan Road, Doha, Qatar

Research and Professional Experience/ Professional Appointments/Honors:

Prof. Dr. Janahi established the section of pediatric pulmonology in 2001 in Qatar and he was acting as the director of pediatric emergency center in parallel from 2001 till 2008. He is currently the section head of pediatric pulmonology at Hamad Medical Corporation (HMC), and the chairman of the national permanent licensing committee (PLC) in the state of Qatar and Professor of Clinical Pediatrics at Weill-Cornell Medical College in Qatar. Prof. Dr. Janahi was a member of the committee that established Qatar's Council for Health Professionals (QCHP), the regulatory body for health practitioners in the state of Qatar. He is also the executive director of Medical Research Center in HMC, and the program director for pediatric residency program with all its educational activities. He is the founder and president of the Gulf Society for Pediatric Respirolgy (GSPR) and a founding member of the Arab Pediatric Pulmonology Association (APPA). He is also a member of the Arab Board examination committee and was instrumental in reforming the Arab Board Pediatric certifying examinations. He sits on advisory boards of few international organizations in the field of pediatric pulmonology and medical education. He also serves on editorial board of few regional and international medical journals.

Publications in Last 3 Years:

1. *Review Article:* Hendaus MA, Janahi IA. Parapneumonic effusion in children: an up-to-date review. *Clin Pediatr* 2016;55(1):10-18.
2. *Editorial Correspondence:* Rehman A, Baloch NU, Janahi IA. Lumacaftor–Ivacaftor in Patients with Cystic Fibrosis Homozygous for Phe508del CFTR. *N Engl J Med* 2015;373(18):1783-1784.
3. *Research Article:* Bhat V, Wahab AA, Garg KC, Janahi IA, Singh R. HRCT in cystic fibrosis in patients with CFTR I1234V mutation: Assessment of scoring systems with low dose technique using multidetector system and correlation with pulmonary function tests. *Indian J Radiol Imaging* 2015;25(1):44-51.
4. *Case Report:* Zahraldin K, Janahi IA, Ben-Omran T, Alsulaiman R, Hamad B, Imam A. Two Qatari siblings with cystic fibrosis and apparent mineralocorticoid excess. *Ann Thorac Med* 2015;10(1):69-72.
5. *Research Article*: Nakkash RT, Al Mulla A, Torossian L, Karhily R, Shuayb L, Mahfoud ZR, Janahi IA, Al Ansari AA, Afifi RA. Challenges to obtaining parental permission for child participation in a school-based waterpipe tobacco smoking prevention intervention in Qatar. *BMC Med Ethics* 2014;15:70.
6. *Research Article:* Molinski SV, Gonska T, Huan LJ, Baskin B, Janahi IA, Ray PN, Bear CE. Genetic, cell biological, and clinical interrogation of the CFTR mutation c.3700 A>G (p.Ile1234Val) informs strategies for future medical intervention. *Genet Med* 2014;16(8):625-632.

In: Cystic and Idiopathic Pulmonary Fibrosis ISBN: 978-1-63485-508-2
Editor: Lorenzo Robertson

Chapter 2

LIVER DISEASE IN CYSTIC FIBROSIS: PREVALENCE, RISK FACTORS, AND OUTCOMES

Fustik Stojka
Center for Cystic Fibrosis, University Children's Clinic,
Skopje, R. Macedonia

ABSTRACT

Liver disease (LD) in cystic fibrosis (CF) has become a matter of greater concern since the population of CF patients lives longer. Early recognition of LD in CF is not easy because its onset is often insidious and clinical, biochemical, and other indicators are relatively insensitive.

Aims: The study analyses the prevalence of CF-related LD in Macedonian CF population and the clinical and genetic characteristics of these patients, in an attempt to find out the possible risk factors for its development.

Methods: All patients older than 2 years (n= 102) were screened for LD through clinical, biochemical, ehographic, and hepatobiliary scintigraphic assessment. LD was defined by the finding of hepatomegaly and/or splenomegaly; significant and persistent increase of at least two serum liver enzyme levels, suggestive ultrasonographic abnormalities (score >4), and morphologic or functional scintigraphic abnormalities.

Results: According to predefined criteria, 33 patients (32.3%) were classified as having LD, three of them with portal hypertension. The clinical presentations of LD had 13, abnormal liver blood test results 21, ultrasound abnormalities 33, and scintigraphic abnormalities 22 of the patients. A male predominance was found in the group with LD (69.7%). Pancreatic insufficiency was present in all patients with LD. There was no significant difference in the pulmonary function, nutritional status, and in the prevalence of meconium ileus or DIOS between groups with and without LD. Genetic analysis showed higher frequency of F508del mutation in LD group (77.3%) vs. no LD group (66.2%). All patients with LD had "severe" mutations: F508del, G542X, N1303K, 621+G→T, R1066C, CFTRdel.21Kb, 1811+1G→C, V456F, R1162X, 457TAT→G, and Y161D.

Conclusion: Male CF patients who have pancreatic insufficiency and carry mutations associated with a severe phenotype are in increased risk to develop LD. Regular screening for LD and identification of patients with liver involvement is of great important in management of CF patients. Our data highlight the value of ultrasound as the most sensitive tool for detection and follow up patents with LD.

Keywords: cystic fibrosis, CFTR gene, liver disease, screening

INTRODUCTION

Although liver cirrhosis was recognized as a complication of cystic fibrosis (CF) in Anderson's original description in 1938, for many years the importance of subclinical liver disease has been eclipsed by the more obvious respiratory and pancreatic signs and symptoms. More effective management of these has resulted in greatly improved survival, and so liver disease (LD) has become important to a large number of CF patients and those involved in their care. Unfortunately, clinical identification of LD in CF is not always easy, because the developing of fibrotic liver lesion is usually clinically silent. Many patients with cirrhosis caused by CF are well compensated and completely asymptomatic and may even have normal liver blood tests. However, with progression of the fibrotic liver lesion, these patients are phone to decompensate and to develop liver failure, requiring liver transplantation. Thus, early diagnosis and therapeutic intervention is important in management of CF patients.

The reported prevalence of LD among CF patients ranges between 9% and 37%, depending on the study and criterion for definition of liver disease [1, 2, 3]. Because there are no sensitive diagnostic markers of liver involvement in CF, the actual prevalence might be even higher. In that context, the postmortem autopsy studies of CF individuals reported that the histological findings of focal biliary cirrhosis were present in 27% of children and 72% of adults [4, 5].

A spectrum of hepatobiliary manifestation observed in CF patients, from mainly asymptomatic elevation of serum liver enzymes, neonatal cholestasis and hepatic steatosis to multilobular cirrhosis and gallbladder abnormalities and approximate frequency of these manifestations are given on table 1 [6, 7].

The pathogenesis of CF associated LD is considered to be secondary effect of the basic defect. The CFTR (cystic fibrosis transmembrane conductance regulator) gene in the normal human liver is expressed in the epithelia of the intrahepatic and extrahepatic bile ducts and gallbladder, and the CFTR protein is localized to the apical domain of these cells [8]. CFTR is not expressed in hepatocytes or other cells of the liver. The proposed pathogenesis of hepatobiliary disease is given by Sokol and Durie [7]. CFTR chloride channel dysfunction caused by CFTR mutations lead to impair or abolish chloride secretion, and concomitant reduction in water and sodium movement into bile. Alter bile composition (hyperviscosity of bile) and decrease bile flow causes obstruction of biliary ducts that may induce collagen synthesis by stellate cells and its deposition in portal tracts in several ways. Defective (sluggish) bile flow cause obstruction of small bile ductules, which is followed by retention of hydrophobic bile acids, exposing the hepatocytes to a high local concentration of potentially toxic bile acid and secondary hepatocyte injure with release of proinflammatory cytokines, growth factors, or lipid peroxide products that recruit and activate hepatic stellate cells to synthesize collagen [9].

Table 1. Hepatobiliary manifestations of CF [6, 7]

Condition	Frequency (%)
Asymptomatic elevation of serum liver enzymes	10-46
Neonatal cholestasis	2
Hepatic steatosis	20-60
Hepatomegaly	30
Focal biliary cirrhosis	10-72
Multilobular cirrhosis	7-20
Cholelithiasis	1-10
Microgallblader	20-30
Common bile duct stenosis	<2

Therefore, obstruction of biliary ducts and bile duct plugging may lead to release of inflammatory mediators, stellate cell activation, collagen deposition in portal tracts, fibrosis, and ultimately, cirrhosis.

The process begins focally in the liver, possibly because of interductal connections that may allow adequate bile drainage of some areas. The progression from cholestasis (decreased bile flow) to focal biliary cirrhosis and to multilobular cirrhosis takes years in some CF patients, or never occurs in other CF patients (Figure 1). The variable onset and severity of LD suggests that there are other genetic or environmental factors (nutritional deficiencies, drug hepatotoxicity, infections, stenosis of the common bile duct by the fibrotic pancreas) that may be involved in the pathogenesis and progression of LD in CF [7, 10, 11].

In biliary cells (cholangiocytes), CFTR appears to play an important role in bile formation and flow. Stimulation of cholangiocyte basolateral receptors by the hormone secretin results in increased intracellular concentration of cAMP, activation of CFTR, and Cl efflux. Efflux of Cl ions from the apical (luminal) membrane generates a lumen-negative potential, which favors movement of Na, and subsequently water into the bile duct lumen.

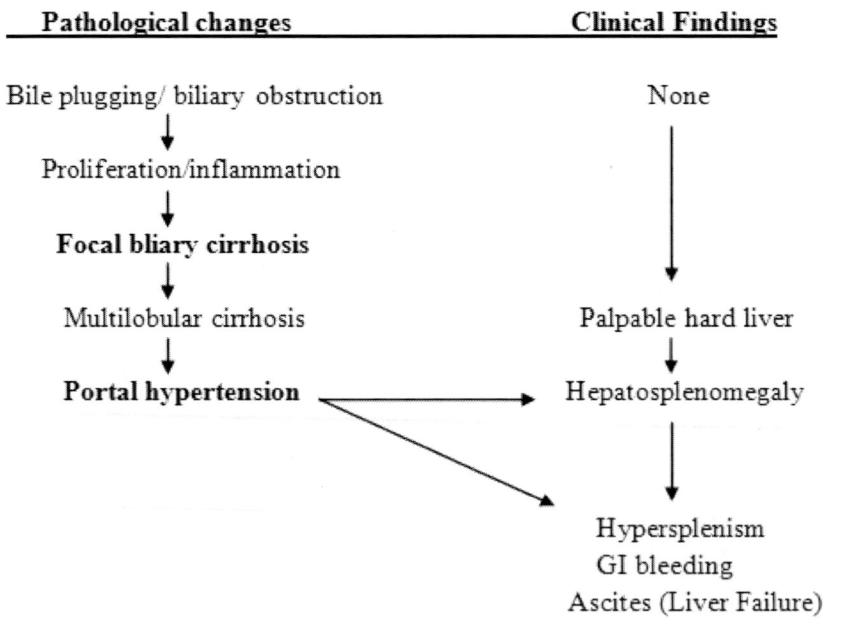

Figure 1. Evolution of liver disease in cystic fibrosis.

Additionally, CFTR regulates HCO_3 transport. Thus, CFTR appears to contribute to normal bile formation and alkalization through the regulation of Cl, HCO3 and water transport. The proposed model by Feranchak implies a prominent role of CFTR in normal bile formation, but it fails to explain why only a select number of patients with CF develop LD despite having abnormal or absent CFTR in bile duct epithelia [6]. Cholangiocytes express several other Cl channels, including G-protein-activated Cl channels, Ca-dependent Cl channels, volume-sensitive Cl channels and Cl channels linked to purinergic receptor stimulation. Although their regulation and contribution to biliary secretion is largely unknown, it is speculate that these alternate Cl conductances may serve to bypass the Cl secretory defect associated with CF.

Only a small fraction (3-5%) of patients with CF develops severe liver disease characterized by cirrhosis with portal hypertension; thus, other modifying genes outside of CF locus disease (non-CFTR genetic variability) may contribute to risk for severe liver disease [12]. Candidate modifying genes, including genes for α_1-antitrypsin or α_1-antiprotease (SERPINA 1), angiotensin-convertin enzyme (ACE), glutathione S-transverase (GSTP1), manose-binding lactin2 (MBL2) and transforming growth factor β1 (TGFB1), have been investigated. It is hypothesize that CF patients are at increased risk for hepatic fibrosis, if they are also carry mutations in other genes pertinent to hepatic inflammation, oxidative stress, or fibrosis. Of these candidate genes, only the SERPINA1 Z allele was significantly associated with CF related LD and portal hypertension [13]. Patients who carry the SERPINA1 Z allele are at greater risk of developing severe LD with portal hypertension. Discoveries in this field may clarify which CF patients are at significant risk for severe LD.

OBJECTIVE

Our study analyses the prevalence of CF-related LD in Macedonian CF population and the clinical and genetic characteristics of these patients, in an attempt to find out the possible risk factors for its development

METHODS

All CF patients older than 2 years (n = 102) who regularly attended the CF Centre at the University Children's Clinic in Skopje, were included in the study. Reports from the sequential screening procedures for LD obtained between 2005-2015 were retrospectively reviewed. Additionally, clinical data and CFTR genotype data of the patients were analyzed.

Screening for Liver Disease

Patients were screened for LD through physical examination, liver biochemistry studies, echographic examination of the upper abdomen, and hepatobiliary scintigraphic assessment.

Physical Examination

Careful examination of liver and spleen was performed at each clinical visit. Hepatomegaly was considered to be present when the edge of the liver was palpable more than 2 cm below the right costal margin; splenomegaly was defined by the finding of palpable spleen below the left costal margin.

Liver Biochemistry Studies

The biochemical evaluation for liver injury and function included serum aspartate aminotransferase (AST), alanine aminotransferase (ALT), gama-glutamyl transpeptidase (GGT), alkaline phosphatase (ALP), and bilirubin level. Liver functional tests were obtained yearly in all CF patients. The results were considered abnormal if at least two serum liver enzyme levels were higher than 1.5 times of the upper limit of normal: AST > 52 IU/L, ALT > 72 IU/L, GGT > 78 IU/L, ALP > 400 IU/L. In those patients the tests were repeated within 3-6 months. If levels remained elevated, without another explanation for the elevation, they were indicative for liver involvement due to CF.

Echographic Examination

Ultrasonography of the liver, biliary tract, gallbladder, spleen and hepatic vasculature was performed yearly in all CF patients older than 2 years. An ultrasound scoring system suggested by Williams et al. [14] was used to provide a grading system for the presence or absence of underlying LD. The scoring system depends upon the detection of three ultrasound characteristics: parenchymal irregularity, periportal fibrosis (increased periportal echoes) and irregularity of the liver edge consistent with the macronodular pattern of cirrhosis (Table 2).

Table 2. The ultrasound scoring system by Williams et al. [14]

Score	1	2	3
Characteristic Hepatic parenchyma Liver edge Periportal fibrosis	 Normal Smooth None	 Coarse - Moderate	 Irregular Nodular Severe

A total score of 3 was consistent with an entirely normal liver (no LD group), while all subjects with a score of 4 or more were allocated in the LD group. The authors suggested that the scoring is able to identify a group of patients with evidence of LD but in pre-cirrhotic phase (score 4-7) and patients with established cirrhosis (score 8 or 9). Doppler ultrasound analysis was used to detect dilatation and flow patterns of hepatic vasculature. Portal hypertension was suggested by enlarged spleen, distended portal vein and abnormal portal venous flow (decreased portal venous flow velocities or reversal of flow).

Hepatobiliary Scintigraphy

Hepatobiliary scintigraphy was performed with brome iminodiacetic acid derivate labeled with technetium–99m (99mTc Mebrofenin). After intravenous administration the derivate is cleared from circulation by hepatocytes, excreted into the canaliculus and bile ducts, stored in the gallbladder, and excreted into the duodenum. 99mTc Mebrofenin was injected intravenously as a bolus. Serial analogue images were taken per frame every 10 seconds for 30 minutes by gamma camera to estimate the dynamic of bile flow, following by static images on 60 and 90 minute. If the gallbladder was seen, the patient was given a high-fat-meal and was subsequently scanned to assess emptying of the gallbladder. If the gallbladder was not seen, additional images were obtained hourly for up to three hours. Morphological scintigraphic abnormalities suggestive for biliary tract obstruction (cholestasis) were: stasis of the tracer in the intrahepatic bile ducts (visualization of secondary and tertiary intrahepatic bile ducts was indicative for intrahpatic delayed excretion); retention of the tracer in the extrahepatic biliary tree; an irregular tapering (segmental narrowing) of the common bile duct; and enlarged gallbladder with delayed emptying. Microgallbladder and not visual gallbladder were relatively frequent scintigraphic findings, but they are not indicative for biliary tract obstruction.

Functional scintigraphic abnormalities suggestive for biliary tract obstruction were: prolonged time of visualization of the intestine (>30 minutes) and prolong half-time of hepatic wash out (normal value: T/2<23 minutes).

Using above mentioned methods, the LD was defined by finding some of these abnormalities: hepatomegaly and/or splenomegaly; significant and persistent increase of at least two serum liver enzyme levels; suggestive ultrasonographic abnormalities (score > 4); and morphologic or functional scintigraphic abnormalities.

Analysis of Clinical and CFTR Genotype Data

The following data from patients' medical history were collected: current age of patient, sex, history of meconium ileus, history of distal intestinal obstruction syndrome (DIOS), pancreatic functional status, current pulmonary function - forced vital capacity (FVC) and forced expiratory volume in the 1st second (FEV_1) expressed as percentage of predicted values and current nutritional status expressed as standard deviation score for height (ZH), standard deviation score for weight (ZW), and body mass index (BMI) for the patients older than 9 years.

Statistic Analysis

The data were analyzed by the Excel Version 9.0 (Microsoft, IL, USA). Variables are reported as means ± SD, unless otherwise stated. Frequency distributions and contingency tables were created for clinical and demographic characteristics of the patients (gender, pancreatic status, meconium ileus or DIOS, liver' variables, and CFTR mutations). Statistical comparisons between two groups of patients with and without LD were performed using Student's t test. The difference was considered significant at $p \leq 0.05$.

RESULTS

Of the 102 CF patients older than 2 years that are regularly followed at CF Center at the University Children's Clinic in Skopje, 33 patients (32.3%) were classified as having CF – related LD, according to predefined criteria. Among them, 13 (39.4%) had clinical signs of LD, 21 (63.6%) had abnormal liver function tests, 22 (66.6%) had scintigraphic abnormalities and all had ultrasonographic changes (Table 3). Abnormal imagines on hepatobiliary scintigraphy were seen in 20 patients and functional scintigraphic abnormalities suggested delayed biliary flow in 7 patients with LD.

Ehographic evidence of hepatic cirrhosis (coarsely nodular liver; score 8 or 9) was found in 17 patients, three of them with portal hypertension (Figure 2). The diagnosis of cirrhosis was confirmed by liver biopsy findings in 7 patients.

Clinical characteristics of the patients with and without LD are reported in Table 4. The prevalence of LD increased with age: average age 13.2±5.3 years in the LD group vs. 9.9±5.6 years in the no LD group. A male predominance was found in the group with LD (69.7%). Pancreatic insufficiency was present in all patients with LD. CF patients with LD tended to have milder pulmonary disease, but the differences in the pulmonary function were not significant. There was also no significant difference in the nutritional status, and in the prevalence of meconium ileus or DIOS between two groups.

Genetic analysis showed higher frequency of F508del mutation in LD group (77.3%) in comparison with no LD group (66.2%), although not statistically significant. Molecular basis of CF in patients with LD is shown in Table 5.

Table 3. Hepatic abnormalities in CF patients with liver disease

Abnormalities	No.	%
Clinical signs of LD	13	39.4
- hepatomegaly	10	30.3
- splenomegaly	3	9.1
Biochemical abnormalities	21	63.6
Ultrasonographic abnormalities	33	100
- ultrasound scor 4-7	19	57.6
- ultrasound scor 8-9 (cirrhosis)	14	42.4
- portal hypertension	3	9.1
Scintigraphic abnormalities	22	66.6
- morphologic	20	60.6
- functional	7	21.2

Table 4. Comparison of clinical variables between patients with and without liver disease

Variables	LD	no LD	p
n (%)	33 (32.3)	69 (67.7)	
Male/female (%)	23/10 (70/30)	39/30 (56/44)	
Current age, years	14.7±5.43	10.91±5.56	<0.05
Pancreatic insufficiency (%)	33 (100)	62 (89.8)	
Meconium ileus/DIOS (%)	1 (3)/4 (12)	3(4.3)/3 (4.3)	
BMI (kg/m^2)	17.6±1.72	16.4±2.58	>0.05
Z-score /Weight	-0.83±1.04	-0.61±0.95	>0.05
Z-score/Height	-0.98±1.44	-0.54±1.15	>0.05
FVC (% predicted)	94.9±14.10	90.38±18.30	>0.05
FEV_1 (% predicted)	90.4±14.83	86.93±22.09	>0.05

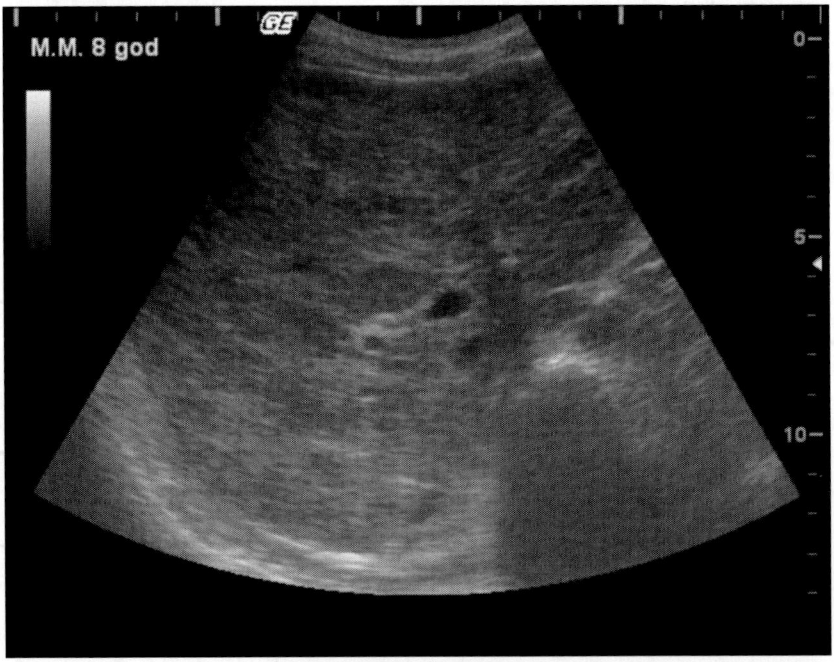

Figure 2. Hepatic ultrasound scan showing marked nodularity (cirrhosis) in 8 years old boy.

Table 5. Genotype frequency in CF patients with liver disease

Genotype	No	%
F508del/F508del	20	60.6
F508del/G542X	2	6
F508del/R1066C	2	6
F508del/V456F	2	6
F508del/621+G→T	1	3
F508del/CFTRdel21	1	3
F508del/457TAT→G	1	3
F508del/1811+1G→C	1	3
F508del//N1303K	1	3
G542X /R1162X	1	3
G542X/Y161D	1	3

All CF patients with LD had "severe" mutations (class I, II or III) associated with pancreatic insufficiency and a more severe clinical course of the disease.

DISCUSSION

Recent advances in the treatment and management of pulmonary complications, development of devoted, multidisciplinary CF clinics and improved modes of nutrition have greatly improved the life expectancy of CF patients. As results, chronic LD has become an important issue among patients with CF and its severity may determine the prognosis of this group. The reported prevalence of liver LD among CF patients varies in different studies. Higher prevalence have been reported in studies in which LD was actively searched for and diagnosed through a combination of diagnostic tools (clinical, biochemical, ultrasonographic evaluation). Long-term follow up of different cohorts of CF patients whose hepatic status was carefully monitored has indicated that the cumulative incidence of liver disease ranges between 27% and 35% [9, 11]. Prevalence seems to increase through childhood into mild-adolescence, with no significant increase thereafter [3]. The large majority of patients in our study developed LD and liver cirrhosis during the first decade of life. This suggests that, for CF patients who will develop liver cirrhosis, the mechanism and risk factors for liver damage are already present in early childhood.

Thus, some patients have progressive LD and develop cirrhosis with portal hypertension and rarely liver insufficiency, while sizeable proportion of patients may have only slight changes that remain stable life-long. Intrinsic abnormalities in the liver of individuals with CF reflect loss of CFTR (Cl^- channel) function on the apical membrane of cholagiocytes. This dysfunction is predict to result in defective (decries) bile flow and is associated with cholangiocytes-inducted inflammatory response with activation and proliferation of hepatic stellate cells, which results in cholangitis and fibrosis in focal portal tracts [7, 9]. Although most CF patients have some degree of liver dysfunction and focal biliary cirrhosis, only 3-5% of CF patients develops severe, end-stage LD [13].

The vast majority of CF patients that develop CF-related LD carry two "severe" (pancreatic insufficient) alleles of CFTR, so it is clear that carrying a mutation with some residual function ("mild", pancreatic sufficient mutations) provides relative protection against the development of the liver cirrhosis. Some authors found LD more often in homozygotes with the most common mutation, F508del, or other mutations associated with pancreatic insufficiency, although studies failed to reveal any relationship with specific CFTR mutations [2, 15, 16]. In our study, the majority of CF patients with LD were F508del homozygous (60.6%) or compound heterozygotes for F508del and other "severe" mutation, associated with complete loss of CFTR function. Only two patients in LD group didn't have F508del mutation on both alleles. All patients in group with LD had pancreatic insufficiency. Thus, our data are in support that patients with pancreatic insufficient and with "severe" CFTR mutations (class I, II, III or VI), especially F508del, are exposed to higher risk for developing LD. LD and especially liver cirrhosis together with pancreatic insufficiency is a component of the severe CF phenotype.

The heterogeneity of phenotype manifestations in individuals with the same CFTR genotypes indicates that disease severity is modulated by other genes and by environmental factors. CF patients with same CFTR genotype, including those homozygous for F508del, exhibit a range of liver involvement, from asymptomatic to severe multilobular cirrhosis with portal hypertension, rarely liver failure. This strongly suggest that non-CFTR genetic factors or possibly environmental factors (nutritional deficiencies, drug hepatotoxicity, infections) may be involved in the pathogenesis and progression of liver disease in CF. A small fraction (~5%) of patients with CF develops severe liver disease characterized by cirrhosis with portal hypertension; thus other modifying genes outside of CF locus are considered to contribute to risk for severe liver disease [12, 13].

To determine the association between non-CFTR genetic polymorphisms and CF-related LD, Bartlett et al. have studied patients with CF and severe liver disease with portal hypertension regarding the presence of 9 functional variants in 5 predefined genes. Of different candidate genes (SERPINA1, ACE, TGFB1, MBL2, GSTP1), only the SERPINA1 Z allele was found to be strongly associated with CF-LD and portal hypertension. The authors concluded that patients who carry the Z allele are at greater risk of developing severe liver disease with portal hypertension [13]. Pereira et al. carried out a study to identify genes associated with hepatic injury and fibrosis in patients with CF- related LD and demonstrated a different expression of several genes associated with hepatic fibrogenesis including, matrix metalloproteinases, collagens and chemokines in patietents with LD versus the control patients, and particularly decreased expression in tissue remodelling genes including tissue inhibitor of metalloproteinase-1 (TIMP-1) and plasminogen activator inhibitor-1 (PAI-1) [17]. These studies show a possible genetic predisposition, independent of the CFTR gene, in the pathogenesis of CFLD, but further data are needed for clarification of this issue.

Liver disease in patients with CF begins insidiously, making it difficult to determine the onset accurately. It seems that the LD usually develops during the first decade and may progress silently, only manifesting as end-stage LD and portal hypertension. Therefore, regular screening for liver disease and identification of patients with the liver involvement, as well as early therapeutic intervention is of great importance in management of CF patients. Screening for liver disease is a part of annual review of patients with CF older than 2-3 years at our center, for many years. The screening includes regular physical examination of liver and spleen, with special attention to the liver span, edge, and consistency; liver functional tests, and annual ultrasonography of the liver, biliary tract, gallbladder, spleen and hepatic vasculature. Hepatobiliary scintigraphy has limited clinical utility compared with ultrasound, but it is useful as an additional method in detecting some morphological and functional abnormalities associated with LD in CF [18]. Liver biopsy may be useful to confirm the presence of LD and determine the extent of portal fibrosis or cirrhosis. However, not all clinicians think that liver biopsy is indicated in investigating LD in CF because the focal pattern of liver involvement which may result in discordance between clinical findings and histological staging, and because patients may be at a higher risk of complications [6, 19].

In the last decade, ultrasound-based elastography methods for non-invasive assessment of chronic liver diseases have been developed. First results of transient elastography (TE) in CF revealed an elevated liver stiffness in patients with CF-related LD [20, 21]. It has been shown that TE could reliably identify children with CFLD and portal hypertension [22]. First data with the recently developed acoustic radiation force impulse imaging (ARFI) technique revealed a high accuracy for the detection of liver cirrhosis in pediatric CF patients with portal hypertension [23]. Magnetic resonance (MR) imaging and MR cholangiopancreatography can be used for the assessment of pancreatic and hepatobiliary complications in CF patients with abdominal symptoms that suggest hepatobiliary involvement [24].

Our study suggested that subclinical LD is common among patients with CF. The criteria for LD in our study were clinical, biochemical, ultrasonografic and radionuclide imaging test results. The physical examination by palpation and measurement of the liver and spleen span below the costal margins should be performed regularly for defining of usually asymptomatic hepatomegaly and/or splenomegaly. Biochemical assessment of liver function would be expected to be the first line investigation. However, previous studies have suggested a low sensitivity and specificity for biochemical indices in the detection of LD in CF and abnormalities usually do not correlate with histological findings [9, 19]. In our study 63.6% of patients in LD group have had evidence of persistent and significant increased liver enzymes during the study period. Our data clearly highlight the value of ultrasound as the most sensitive tool for detection and follow up patents with LD. Ultrasonographic abnormalities of liver appearance were more frequent than biochemical abnormalities, and once present were more likely to be persistent. The ultrasound scoring system suggested by Williams et al. [14] is, we believe, simple and useful for detection, grading and monitoring the progression of LD. For better assessment of hepatic status, hepatobiliary scintigraphy was performed in patients with suggestive ultrasonographic abnormalities. We found that radionuclide imaging test provides useful information about liver function and biliary secretion and could be added in the screening methods for identification of LD and for monitoring the response to therapy. Liver biopsy and hystologic assessment of liver was not included in the study protocol. Needle biopsies of the liver were performed only in several patients. The widespread use of an invasive technique, with an attendant risk of haemorrhage, is probably not acceptable, especially within the pediatric population.

Implementation of screening program for liver disease is an important step in targeting population for early intervention and prophylactic treatment. At present, oral ursodeoxycholic acid (UDCA) therapy, aimed at improving billiary secretion in terms of bile viscosity and bile composition, is the only available therapeutic approach in CF-related LD. UDCA, a naturally occurring hydrophilic bile acid, has in many studies been shown to normalize liver enzymes, improve hepatobiliary scintigraphy and suggested an improvement in liver morphology [25, 26, 27, 28], but so far an effect of UDCA on the ultimate outcome of the disease has not yet be proven. However, there evidence suggests that the use of UDCA at an early stage may abort or inhibit the development of LD in CF, thus may favorably affect the natural course of the focal billiary fibrosis/cirrhosis [26, 28].

In CF patients who develop cirrhosis, it is necessary to screen for complications related to portal hypertension (e.g., esophageal or gastric varices, hepatopulmonary and portopulmonary syndromes) and for signs of liver failure. Management should focus mainly on nutrition, prevention of bleeding and variceal decompression. Liver transplantation is a treatment of choice for patients with the advanced CF-related LD and preserved pulmonary function (FEV1>50%) [29]. The indication for liver transplantation considered a variety of factors including liver failure, hypersplenism, malnutrition, gastro-esophageal bleeding, and worsening pulmonary function [29, 30]. Two scoring systems evaluating the need for transplantation are available, both of which include and parameters of nutritional status [31, 32]. Most authors suggest that liver transplantation should be performed prior to the development of end-stage liver disease or overt pulmonary or other clinical decompensation [29]. Clear indications for liver transplantation in CF liver disease are [11]:

- progressive hepatic dysfunction (falling albumin <30 g/l; increasing coagulopathy, not corrected by vitamin K)
- development of ascites and jaundice
- intractable variceal bleeding which is not controlled by conventional means
- hepatopulmonary and portopulmonary syndromes
- severe malnutrition, unresponsive to intensive nutritional support
- deteriorating quality of life related to LD
- deteriorating pulmonary function (FEV1/FVC <50%).

The transplant assessment should evaluate pulmonary and cardiac function in order to establish whether liver transplantation alone is required or a combined heart/lung/liver transplant is more appropriate.

CONCLUSION

Early recognition of LD in CF is not easy because its onset is often insidious and the clinical, biochemical and other indicators are relatively insensitive. It has been suggested that early therapy may prevent progression of CF-related LD. Implementation of screening program for LD in all CF patients older than 2-3 years is an important step in targeting population for early intervention and prophylactic treatment. The policy for examining only patients with abnormal liver function test results or those who are symptomatic, fails to detect a number of young patients who clearly have abnormal eho texture to the liver, some of whom may progress to more severe LD. UDCA therapy may have the greatest benefit if initiated early in the course of the disease, prior to the development of focal biliary cirrhosis and multilobular cirrhosis, again emphasizing the need for sensitive and specific markers for early detection of CFLD. Patients identified by screening procedures are expected to progress at a slower rate than patients who first came to attention as a result of symptoms. Therefore, active follow-up evaluation directed at detection of LD should be started early in the life, preferentially in patients with mail gender, pancreatic insufficient and with severe CFTR mutations, who are exposed to higher risk for developing this complication of CF.

REFERENCES

[1] Scott-Jupp R., Lama M., Tanner M. S. Prevalence of liver disease in cystic fibrosis. *Arch. Dis. Child.,* 1991; 66:698–701.

[2] Wilschanski M., Rivlin J., Cohen S., et al. Clinical and genetic risk factors for cystic fibrosis-related liver disease. *Pediatrics,* 1999; 103: 52-8.

[3] Colombo C., Battezzati P. M., Crosignani A., et al. Liver disease in cystic fibrosis: a prospective study on incidence, risk factors and outcome. *Hepatology*, 2002; 36:1374–82.

[4] Oppenheimer E. H., Esterly J. R. Hepatic changes in young infants with cystic fibrosis: possible relation to focal biliary cirrhosis. *J. Pediatr.*, 1975; 86:683-9.

[5] Vawter G. F., Shwachman H. Cystic fibrosis in adults: an autopsy study. *Pathol. Ann.*, 1979; 14:357-82.

[6] Feranchak A. P. Hepatobiliary complications of cystic fibrosis. *Curr. Gastroenterol. Rep.*, 2004; 6:231-9.

[7] Sokol R. J., Durie P. R. Recommendations for management of liver and biliary tract disease in cystic fibrosis. Cystic Fibrosis Foundation Hepatobiliary Disease Consensus Group. *J. Pediatr. Gastroenterol. Nutr.*, 1999; 28(Suppl. 1):1–13.

[8] Cohn J. A., Strong T. V., Picciotto M. R., et al. Localization of the cystic fibrosis transmembrane conductance regulator in human bile duct epithelial cells. *Gastroenterology,* 1993; 105:1857-64.

[9] Colombo C. Liver disease in cystic fibrosis. *Curr. Opin. Pulm. Med.,* 2007; 13:529-36.

[10] Moyer K., Balisteri W. Hepatobiliary disease in patients with cystic fibrosis. *Curr. Opin. Gastroenterol.*, 2009; 25:272-8.

[11] Debray D., Kelly D., Houwen R., Strandvik B., Colombo C. Best practice guidance for the diagnosis and management of cystic fibrosis associated liver disease. *J. Cyst. Fibros.,* 2011; 10(Suppl. 2):S29-S36.

[12] Castaldo G., Fuccio A., Salvatore D., et al. Liver expression in cystic fibrosis could be modulated by genetic factors different from the cystic fibrosis transmembrane regulator genotype. *Am. J. Med. Genet.,* 2001; 98:294-7.

[13] Bartlett J. R., Friedman K. J., Ling S., et al.; for the Gene Modifier Study Group. Genetic modifiers of liver disease in cystic fibrosis. *JAMA,* 2009; 302:1076-83.

[14] Williams S. G., Evanson J. E., Barrett N., et al. An ultrasound scoring system for the diagnosis of liver disease in cystic fibrosis. *J. Hepatol.,* 1995; 22:513-21.

[15] De Arce M., O'Brien S., Hegarty J., et al. Deletion F508 and clinical expression of cystic fibrosis-related liver disease. *Clin. Genet.,* 1992; 42:271-2.

[16] Wilschanski M., Durie P. R. Patterns of GI disease in adulthood associated with mutations in the CFTR gene. *Gut,* 2007; 56:1153-63.

[17] Pereira T. N., Lewindon P. J., Greer R. M., et al. Transcriptional basis for hepatic fibrosis in cystic fibrosis-associated liver disease. *J. Pediatr. Gastroenterol. Nutr.*, 2012; 54(3):328-35.

[18] O'Connor P. J., Sounthern K. W., Bowler I. M., et al. The role of hepatic scintigraphy in cystic fibrosis. *Hepatology,* 1996; 23: 281-7.

[19] Potter C. J., Fishbein M., Hammond S., et al. Can the histologic changes of cystic fibrosis-associated hepatobiliary disease be predicted by clinical criteria? *J. Pediatr. Gastroenterol. Nutr.*, 1997; 25: 32-6.

[20] Menten R., Leonard A., Clapuyt P., et al. Transient elastography in patients with cystic fibrosis. *Pediatr. Radiol.,* 2010; 40: 1231–5.

[21] Witters P., Boeck K. de, Dupont L., et al. Non-invasive liver elastography (Fibroscan) for detection of cystic fibrosisassociated liver disease. *J. Cyst. Fibros.*, 2009; 8: 392–9.

[22] Malbrunot-Wagner A. C., Bridoux L., Nousbaum J. B., et al. Transient elastography and portal hypertension in pediatric patients with cystic fibrosis. *J. Cyst. Fibros.,* 2011; 10:338–42.

[23] Manco M., Lo Zupone C., Latini A., et al. Noninvasive assessment of cystic fibrosis-associated liver disease with acoustic radiation force impulse imaging. *Hepatology,* 2011; 53: 1779–80.

[24] King L. J., Scurr E. D., Murugan N., et al. Hepatobiliary and pancreatic manifestations of cystic fibrosis: MR imaging appearances. *Radiographics,* 2000; 20(3):767-77.

[25] Colombo C., Battezzati P. M., Padda M., et al. Ursodeoxycholic acid for liver disease associated with cystic fibrosis: a double-blind multicenter trial. *Hepatology,* 1996; 23: 1484-90.

[26] Linblad A., Glaumann H., Strandvik B. A two-year prospective study of the effect of ursodeoxycholic acid on urinary bile acid excretion and liver morphology in cystic fibrosis- associated liver disease. *Hepatology,* 1998; 27: 166-74.

[27] Fustik S., Josifovska T., Pop-Jordanova N., et al. Liver disease in cystic fibrosis. *Contributions, Sec. Bilol. Med. Sci.,* 2000; XXI/1-2: 29-40.

[28] Nausia-Avranitakis S., Fountoulaki M., Economou H., et al. A. Long-term prospective study of the effect of ursodeoxycholic acid on cystic fibrosis related liver disease. *J. Clin. Gastroenterol.,* 2001; 32: 324-8.

[29] Melzi M. J., Kelly D. A., Colombo C., et al. Liver transplantation in cystic fibrosis: a poll among European centers. A study from the European Liver Transplant Registry. *Transpl. Int.,* 2006; 19:726-31.

[30] Nash K. L., Collier J. D., French J., et al. Cystic fibrosis liver disease: to transplant or not to transplant? Am. J. Transplant., 2008; 8:162-9.

[31] Noble-Jamieson G., Barnes N., Jamieson N., et al. Liver transplantation for hepatic cirrhosis in cystic fibrosis. *J. Royal. Soc. Med.,* 1996;89: 31–7.

[32] Milkiewicz P., Skiba G., Kelly D., et al. Transplantation for cystic fibrosis: outcome following early liver transplantation. *J. Gastroenterol. Hepatol.,* 2002; 17:208.

In: Cystic and Idiopathic Pulmonary Fibrosis
Editor: Lorenzo Robertson
ISBN: 978-1-63485-508-2

Chapter 3

LUNG TRANSPLANTATION FOR CYSTIC FIBROSIS

Zubin Mukadam[1], MD, Mehgan Holland[2], BS and Keith C. Meyer[1,*], MD, MS

[1]Department of Medicine, University of Wisconsin School of Medicine and Public Health, Madison, WI, US

[2]Division of Pulmonary and Critical Care Medicine, University of Wisconsin School of Medicine and Public Health, Madison, WI and the Department of Surgery, Division of Cardiothoracic Surgery, University of Wisconsin School of Medicine and Public Health, Madison, WI, US

ABSTRACT

Although the benefits of lung transplantation for young children with cystic fibrosis (CF) remains somewhat controversial, lung transplantation is the only therapeutic option that is likely to improve survival and quality of life for children and adult patients with CF who have advanced bronchiectatic lung disease and progressive respiratory failure that is

* Corresponding author: Keith C. Meyer, MD, MS, FACP, FCCP. Professor of Medicine, University of Wisconsin Lung Transplant and Advanced Lung Disease Program, Section of Allergy, Pulmonary and Critical Care Medicine, Department of Medicine, University of Wisconsin School of Medicine and Public Health, tel: 608 263-6363 (office), 608 263-3035 (secretary); fax: 608 263-3104; e-mail: kcm@medicine.wisc.edu.

unresponsive to other therapies. If patients wish to be candidates for lung transplantation, the appearance of signs of impending respiratory failure should trigger referral to a transplant center where a lung transplant team can determine whether criteria for lung transplantation are met and whether potential recipients lack absolute contraindications for transplantation. Major obstacles to long-term survival of lung transplant recipients include peri-operative complications, infections, and the development of chronic lung allograft dysfunction (CLAD). However, despite the many potential complications of lung transplantation, recipients can have prolonged survival and good quality of life. This chapter reviews referral criteria, contraindications to lung transplantation, and candidate evaluation and listing. Additionally, technical aspects of donor lung implantation, principles of peri-operative and post-transplant management, and long-term outcomes are discussed.

Keywords: lung transplantation, cystic fibrosis

INTRODUCTION

Advances in our understanding of CF and the development of therapies to improve nutrition, clear infected secretions from the lungs, treat and/or prevent acute exacerbations of chronic lung disease, and suppress chronic lung infections and inflammation have substantially prolonged the survival of patients with CF such that median survival has increased from approximately 10 years of age in 1960 to nearly 39 years in 2016. Our identification and understanding of abnormal variants of the dysfunctional CF transmembrane regulator (CFTR) protein that is produced from mutant CFTR genes combined with the introduction of modulators that can improve intracellular production and function of the CFTR protein may also have a significant, genotype-dependent impact on the progressively worsening bronchiectatic lung disease that eventually leads to respiratory failure. Despite these evolving advances in care and greatly improved survival over the past few decades, most patients will eventually develop end-stage lung disease and qualify for lung transplantation, which can substantially improve quality of life (QOL) and extend survival for patients who would otherwise succumb to death due to respiratory failure.

Although most patients now survive to adulthood with relatively few needing lung transplantation as children, cystic fibrosis remains the most common indication for lung transplantation in the pediatric population and accounts for 70-75% of transplants in pediatric patients. However, because

CFTR dysfunction affects not only the respiratory tract but also the pancreas, biliary tract, gastrointestinal tract, and paranasal sinuses, a substantial percentage of adult patients with CF will have CF-related diabetes, hepatic dysfunction, chronic sinusitis, and other CF-related co-morbidities. Additionally, the burden of coping with chronic disease leads to clinical depression and anxiety in nearly one-third of adult patients, compliance/ adherence to prescribed therapies is often suboptimal, and access to newly available pharmacologic treatments such as ivacaftor and combined ivacaftor/ lumacaftor may be limited.

After the indications of fibrotic lung disease and chronic obstructive pulmonary disease (COPD), end-stage lung disease due to CF is the third most common indication for lung transplantation. This chapter reviews referral criteria, patient selection, pre- and post-transplant management, complications, and long-term outcomes for patients with advanced CF lung disease.

SELECTION OF PATIENTS FOR LUNG TRANSPLANTATION

Criteria for Referral

A key trigger for referral to a lung transplant center is a persistent decline in forced expiratory volume in one second (FEV1) to less than 30% of the predicted normal value (Table 1). Other indications for referral include a rapid decline in FEV1 (especially for female patients), the development of pulmonary arterial hypertension, a decline in walk distance to <400 m during a 6-minute walk test (6-MWT), or a decline in clinical status that is characterized by increasing bacterial resistance to antibiotics and poor recovery from respiratory exacerbations, worsening nutritional status despite nutritional supplementation, an episode of pneumothorax or life-threatening hemoptysis despite undergoing bronchial artery embolization, or an episode of respiratory failure that requires assisted ventilation.

Waiting times for children, especially if small, are longer than those for adults. Therefore, children should be referred as early as possible when the following are present: (1) short predicted life expectancy; (2) progressive lung disease despite maximal medical therapy; (3) poor quality of life. An adequate support system should be in place, and the child, if possible, should commit to the transplantation procedure and all required aspects of post-transplant long-term follow-up. Also, because non-adherence to required therapies is a leading cause of lung allograft dysfunction in adolescent recipients, the consequences of potential non-adherence to post-transplant therapies should be addressed when transplant candidacy is initially assessed.

Table 1. Lung Transplant for CF: Guidelines for Referral and Transplantation*

Criteria for referral:

- FEV1 <30% or rapid decline in FEV1 despite optimal therapy (especially young females)
- 6-MWT distance <400 m
- Development of PH (systolic PAP >35 mm Hg on echo or mean PAP >25 mm Hg on RHC)
- Clinical decline characterized by increasing frequency of exacerbations and:
  - Episode of respiratory failure requiring non-invasive ventilation
  - Increasing antibiotic resistance and poor clinical recovery from exacerbations
  - Worsening nutritional status despite supplementation
  - Pneumothorax
  - Life-threatening hemoptysis despite bronchial embolization

Criteria for listing for transplantation:

- Chronic respiratory failure
  - With hypoxia alone (PaO2 <60 mm Hg)
  - With hypercapnia (PaCO2 >50 mm Hg)
- Long-term non-invasive ventilation therapy
- Pulmonary hypertension
- Frequent hospitalization
- Rapid lung function decline
- WHO Functional Class IV

* Based on expert opinion consensus (Weill D et al. J Heart Lung Transplant. 2015; 34:1-15).

Abbreviations: FEV1 = forced expiratory volume in one second; 6-MWT = six-minute walk test; PAP = pulmonary artery pressure; PH = pulmonary hypertension; RHC = right heart catheterization; WHO = world health organization.

Contraindications

There are many absolute contraindications that should be considered prior to or at the time of referral (Table 2). Contraindications that are particularly important issues for patients with CF include a history of non-adherence to medical therapies and lack of an adequate social support system. Although mechanical ventilation is a relative contraindication, patients who are otherwise stabilized and have no other contraindications to transplant can do as well as patients who do not require invasive ventilatory support. Another relative contraindication is infection with organisms that are highly resistant to antibiotic therapy (*Burkholderia cenocepacia, Burkholderia gladioli*, and multi-drug–resistant *Mycobacterium abscessus*). Poorer outcomes (significantly decreased survival) have been observed by a number of centers for patients infected with *B. gladioli* or *B. cenocepacia*, and these patients should be referred to centers that are willing to transplant such patients and have experience in the management of patients with chronic *B. cepacia* complex infection. Similarly, because the non-tuberculous mycobacterium (NTM), *M. abscessus*, has also been associated with invasive and refractory post-transplant infections, many centers are reluctant to transplant patients who have evidence of chronic colonization/infection with this microorganism, although an appreciable effect on survival has not been demonstrated. However, chronic infection with other resistant bacteria, such as *Pseudomonas aeruginosa* or methicillin-resistant *Staphylococcus aureus* (MRSA), is more amenable to medical management, and chronic colonization/infection with multi-drug resistant P. aeruginosa or other bacteria such as *Stenotrophomonas* or *Achromobacter* species in their secretions does not appear to have a significant impact on short or long-term outcomes. Infections with other NTM species (e.g., M. avium complex) is also usually manageable with appropriate anti-mycobacterial antibiotic therapy. Fungal colonization with *Aspergillus* species can be detected in over half of adult CF patients prior to lung transplantation but does not appear to be associated with worse short-term mortality. However, significant post-transplant infections can occur, especially anastomotic infections with *A. fumigatus*. Some centers have reported a significant impact of *Aspergillus* colonization on longer term mortality, and prophylactic inhaled nebulized amphotericin B and an imidazole (e.g., itraconazole, voriconazole) is given post-operatively at our center and maintained until anastomoses are completely healed and surveillance studies no longer detect persistent fungal infection.

Table 2. Contraindications to Lung Transplantation

Absolute contraindications
▪ Malignancy (5-year disease-free interval required except for non-melanoma skin cancer)
▪ Untreatable advanced dysfunction of another major organ system (combined organ transplant may be an option)
▪ Uncorrected atherosclerotic disease
▪ Acute medical instability
▪ Uncorrectable bleeding diathesis
▪ Chronic infection with highly virulent and/or resistant microbes that are poorly controlled prior to transplant
▪ Active *Mycobacterium tuberculosis* infection
▪ Significant chest wall or spinal deformity that is expected to cause severe restriction after transplantation
▪ BMI $\geq$35 kg/m^2 (class 2 or 3 obesity)
▪ Non-adherence to medical therapy
▪ Psychiatric conditions associated with inability to cooperate with the health care team and/or adhere with complex medical therapies
▪ Absence of an adequate or reliable social support system
▪ Severely limited functional status with poor rehabilitation potential
▪ Substance abuse or dependence
Relative contraindications
▪ Age >65 years (>75 years unlikely to be candidates in most cases)
▪ Class I obesity (BMI 30-34.9 kg/m^2, especially if central/truncal)
▪ Progressive or severe malnutrition
▪ Severe, symptomatic osteoporosis
▪ Extensive prior chest surgery with lung resection
▪ Mechanical ventilation and/or ECLS (however, carefully selected candidates without other acute or chronic organ dysfunction may be successfully transplanted)
▪ Colonization or infection with highly resistant or highly virulent bacteria, fungi, and certain strains of mycobacteria (e.g., chronic extrapulmonary infection expected to worsen after transplantation).
▪ Hepatitis B or C
▪ HIV infection
▪ Infection with *Burkholderia cenocepacia*, *Burkholderia gladioli*, and multi-drug–resistant *Mycobacterium abscessus*
▪ Atherosclerotic disease with end-organ risk
▪ Other serious medical conditions without end-stage organ damage (e.g., diabetes, HTN, epilepsy, PUD/GER, etc.)

Abbreviations: BMI = body mass index; ECLS = extracorporeal life support; HTN = systemic hypertension; PUD = peptic ulcer disease; GER = gastroesophageal reflux.

Pre-Transplant Evaluation

Candidates for lung transplantation must be carefully evaluated to ensure that no absolute contraindications exist and to consider relative contraindications, such as significant psychosocial issues, the presence of poorly controlled diabetes with significant end-organ damage, active infection associated with a significantly increased likelihood of poor outcomes, or unstable condition in an intensive care unit setting (Table 3). A comprehensive psychosocial evaluation should be performed that includes whether patients have complied with medical therapies, use tobacco or abuse drugs, have a history of significant psychiatric illness, and whether they have adequate social support. A comprehensive cardiopulmonary evaluation with pulmonary function testing, a 6-MWT, appropriate thoracic imaging (including measurement of thoracic cage dimensions), electrocardiogram, echocardiogram, and right heart catheterization should be performed. Additional components of candidate evaluation include routine laboratory testing (e.g., metabolic profile with glucose, creatinine, and blood urea nitrogen, complete blood count, and liver function testing), an infection-specific evaluation (sputum bacterial and mycobacterial cultures), and bone mineral density measurement. Other testing can be considered, such as pH/impedance testing to detect pathologic gastroesophageal reflux and colonoscopy to detect colonic neoplastic lesions.

The decision to proceed with lung transplantation must especially consider extrapulmonary manifestations of CF, infectious disease history, and degree of pulmonary function impairment. Severe malnutrition (e.g., BMI <18) is a concern, but whether this has a significant impact on outcomes for patients with CF is not entirely clear. If potential candidates have significant liver or renal disease that is likely to compromise outcomes following lung transplantation, a multi-organ transplant by centers experienced with such procedures should be considered.

Table 3. Pre-transplant evaluation of referred patients

▪ Ensure that no absolute contraindications exist
▪ Thoroughly consider relative contraindications
▪ Comprehensive psychosocial evaluation (performed by transplant social worker)
– Compliance with medical therapies?
– Use of tobacco?
– Drug abuse (illicit drugs, narcotics)?

Table 3. (Continued)

- – History of significant psychiatric illness?
- – Adequate social support system in place?
- – Psychiatric evaluation if needed
- ▪ Cardiopulmonary evaluation
  - – Pulmonary evaluation
    - · Pulmonary function testing
    - · 6-MWT
    - · Appropriate thoracic imaging
    - · Routine chest x-ray (measurement of thoracic cage dimensions)
    - · Thoracic high-resolution computed tomography scan
    - · Quantitative ventilation/perfusion lung scan
  - – Cardiac evaluation
    - · Electrocardiogram and echocardiogram
    - · Right heart catheterization (consider left heart catheterization with coronary angiography in patients >45 yrs of age or if risk factors for CAD are present)
- ▪ Laboratory testing
  - – Routine laboratory testing
    - · Metabolic profile with glucose, electrolytes, creatinine, and blood urea nitrogen
    - · Complete blood count
    - · Liver function testing, fasting lipid profile
    - · Urinalysis
  - – Special tests
    - · Viral serologies (HIV, CMV, EBV, VZV, HBsAg, HBsAb, HCV, HSV)
    - · Toxoplasma antibody
    - · Blood type and screen
    - · Panel reactive antibody and specific anti-HLA antibody screening
- ▪ Infection specific evaluation (sputum bacterial and mycobacterial cultures, tuberculosis screening)
- ▪ Bone densitometry
- ▪ Nutritional screening (performed by a nutritionist)
- ▪ Dental evaluation
- ▪ Ophthalmologic evaluation
- ▪ Cancer screening as appropriate for age and gender
- ▪ Other testing if appropriate
  - – Contrast esophagram ± pH/impedance testing to detect pathologic gastroesophageal reflux
  - – Colonoscopy to detect colonic neoplastic lesions

Abbreviations: CMV = cytomegalovirus; EBV = Epstein-Barr virus; HBsAb = hepatitis B surface antibody; HBsAb = hepatitis B surface antibody; HCV = hepatitis C virus; HIV = human immunodeficiency virus; HSV = Herpes simplex virus; VZV = Varicella zoster virus; 6-MWT = 6-minute walk test.

Listing for Transplantation

Key observations or events that indicate that patients should be listed for lung transplant include rapid decline in lung function, frequent hospitalization, the presence of pulmonary hypertension, progression to World Health Organization (WHO) Functional Class IV, need for long-term, non-invasive ventilation, and/or chronic respiratory failure as reflected by significant hypoxemia with arterial partial pressure of oxygen (PaO_2) <60 mm Hg or partial pressure of carbon dioxide (PaCO2) >50 mm Hg (Table 1). Patients with CF are universally listed for bilateral sequential lung transplant (to avoid leaving a septic native lung in place as would be the case if a single lung procedure was performed), and the majority of donor lungs come from donors who have suffered brain death. However, lungs may be available from deceased donors who undergo controlled cardiac death, and living-related lobar donation is occasionally performed. Prioritization on the waiting list is determined in the United States by the Lung Allocation Scoring (LAS) system, which balances medical urgency for transplantation (the predicted risk that a patient will die within one year) with the estimated transplant benefit (the number of additional days of life expected during the first post-transplant year if the patient receives a lung transplant). Multivariate regression models that analyze various predictors are used to generate an LAS value (ranging from 0 to 100) that is derived from the output of these models. Priority is generally given to waitlisted patients with a higher score who are matched to a donor by blood type and thoracic cage dimensions.

The use of donation after cardiac death (DCD) donors (non-heart-beating donors who have undergone planned and controlled withdrawal of life support) has provided an additional pool of donated organs as an alternative to the traditional brain-dead donor. Reports in the literature indicate that recipient outcomes are similar to those for lungs transplanted from brain-dead donors, and using DCD donors can help expand the pool of donor lungs available for transplant. Additionally, *ex vivo* lung perfusion (EVLP) has recently emerged as a technique that can be used to evaluate and recondition lungs that have been explanted from a donor such that the function of marginal/injured lungs can be evaluated and potentially improved over an 18-48 hour time period such that significant dysfunction can be avoided if such donor lungs are then found to have adequate function and can be transplanted into a recipient.

Transplanting patients who are receiving life support in the intensive care unit and the use of extracorporeal membrane oxygenation (ECMO) to support patients with severe respiratory failure has gradually increased, but outcomes for patients on either mechanical ventilation or ECMO have been significantly inferior when compared to recipients who do not require such support. Nonetheless, ECMO may provide the only means of keeping a patient alive for transplantation and can also be used to support recipients through the transplant procedure. However, patients with CF receiving assisted or invasive ventilator support who are otherwise free of other contraindications to lung transplant can have outcomes that are not inferior to patients with CF who do not require such ventilator support prior to transplantation.

Preparation for Transplantation

Management of CF (both pulmonary and extra-pulmonary manifestations of disease) should be optimized to maximize the likelihood of peri- and intraoperative stability and optimal longer term outcomes. Because post-transplant infections are a leading cause of morbidity and mortality for recipients with CF and the bronchiectatic lungs of CF patients are chronically infected with bacteria (e.g., *P. aeruginosa*, *S. aureus*) that are often antibiotic-resistant, a 10- to 14-day course of empiric intravenous antibiotics (formulated prior to the transplant event in consultation with a transplant infectious disease consultant and with double-coverage whenever possible) that is tailored to organisms isolated from a recent pre-transplant sputum specimen is initiated at the time of transplant for all recipients with CF at our center. The antibiotic regimen is adjusted within 24-48 hours of transplant according to bacterial isolates and their antibiotic susceptibilities from bronchial aspirates obtained when the native lungs are explanted. Similarly, because paranasal sinuses are chronically infected and drainage into the nasopharynx is usually obstructed due to chronic inflammation and mucosal thickening that compromises ostia, patients are evaluated by an otolaryngologist who specializes in sinus issues and sinus surgery, and endoscopic sinus surgery is performed if needed to promote drainage of paranasal sinuses.

In addition to standard-of-care treatment of chronic lung disease, other common manifestations of CF must be adequately managed. CF-related diabetes (CFRD), osteopenia/osteoporosis, various potential gastrointestinal issues, and neuropsychiatric disorders (anxiety and depression) are common in adult patients with CF. Additionally, the prevalence of CFRD (often linked to corticosteroid and immunosuppressive therapies used in post-transplant maintenance immunosuppression regimens), bone demineralization with compression fractures, and significant gastroesophageal reflux (GER) typically increases post-transplant. Insulin may be required for treatment of CFRD, vitamin D and bisphosphonates may be needed for osteoporosis/osteopenia, and medical and/or surgical (anti-reflux surgery with fundoplication) may be needed to treat GER disease (GERD) and the potential it poses for post-transplant allograft function should GER and lower respiratory tract aspiration occur. Patients may have significant biliary dysfunction, and distal intestinal obstruction (DIOS) may occur in the post-transplant setting. The risk of DIOS can be reduced by appropriate pre- and post-transplant bowel regimens used to prevent intestinal obstruction.

Surgical Issues and Technical Considerations

Because of the perceived risk of leaving a single native lung that harbors chronic bacterial infection in the chest should a single lung transplant be performed on a patient with CF, virtually all patients undergo a bilateral sequential lung transplant, and heart-lung transplants, while frequently performed in the 1980s and early 1990s for patients with CF are no longer performed. Lobar transplants are occasionally performed for recipients with small chests, and lobar transplants from two living-related donors (e.g., one lower lobe each from mother and father) are occasionally performed in centers with expertise in this procedure.

Because many patients with CF have had pneumothoraces, pleural infections (and may have had pleurodesis), lung tissue resections (e.g., for recurrent hemoptysis), or adhesed and neovascularized pleurae, explanting the native lungs can be quite challenging and difficult when surgical removal is attempted. A "clamshell" incision that gives excellent access to pleural spaces is a preferred approach, and some centers prefer to use cardiopulmonary bypass (CPB) during the procedure, although closed extracorporeal membrane oxygenation circuits are now being used by many centers and may lower the risk of bleeding from higher amounts of heparin required for CPB procedures. At our center, aggressive bronchoscopic clearance of the recipient's native lungs is performed following intubation (using a double-lumen tube) to diminish risk of soiling the surgical field with infected secretions. Saline that contains tobramycin is used for bronchoscopic irrigation, and secretion clearance facilitates single lung ventilation during the first stages of a bilateral sequential lung transplant and adequate single lung ventilation can decrease CBP time required and the risk of bleeding due to prolonged anticoagulation. Secretion aspiration via a suction catheter that is maintained in a position such that secretions from the first native explanted lung can be cleared when such secretions are propelled proximally during native lung manipulation and dissection. This is also done as the second native lung is manipulated, dissected, and explanted. Bilateral large bore chest tubes are placed as implantation is completed and left in place until the pleural spaces are determined to be clear of infection and have minimal output.

POST-TRANSPLANT MANAGEMENT

Peri-Operative Management and Complications

Major early complications that affect allograft function include surgical site complications, primary graft dysfunction (PGD) that represents ischemia/reperfusion acute lung injury that occurs within 48-72 hrs post-implantation and significantly impairs early graft function, infection, and hyperacute rejection (usually caused by recipient pre-formed anti-human leukocyte antigen [HLA] antibodies that recognize donor lung alloantigens) (Table 4). Appropriate/optimal surgical technique, immunosuppression, and infection prophylaxis are key to maximal and sustained allograft function. Subacute allograft dysfunction is usually caused by infection or non-infectious acute lung allograft dysfunction (ALAD), which is frequently caused by acute cellular rejection (ACR). If an acute post-transplant complication (e.g., untreated infection) is suspected, a diagnosis must be aggressively sought, and appropriate treatment, which may need to be empiric initially, must be started as soon as possible. Imaging studies (computed tomography, ultrasound, etc.) can be invaluable in making a prompt diagnosis. Infections can arise in the lung allografts, pleural spaces, wound sites, or extrapulmonary sites (e.g., intravenous catheters, indwelling infusaports that have not been removed) and remain a constant threat to lung transplant recipients. In addition to peri- and post-operative antibacterial antibiotics, a prophylactic regimen (intravenous ganciclovir that is eventually transitioned to valganciclovir) to suppress cytomegalovirus (CMV) infection is given to all recipients at our center and has greatly reduced the impact of CMV disease on recipient survival. Similarly, chronic prophylactic therapy (e.g., trimethoprim sulfmethoxazole) is given to prevent *Pneumocystic jiroveci* pneumonia, and chronic prophylactic/ suppressive therapy (e.g., acyclovir, valacyclovir) is given to prevent *Herpes simplex* virus infections.

Table 4. Complications of Lung Transplantation

Pulmonary Complications
▪ Complications affecting the allograft(s)
– Primary graft dysfunction (PGD)
– Surgical complications
– Rejection (hyperacute, acute cellular, antibody-mediated)
– Neutrophilic reversible allograft dysfunction (NRAD)
– Chronic lung allograft dysfunction (CLAD)
· Obstructive BOS
· Restrictive allograft syndrome (RAS)
· Multi-factorial
– Anastomosis abnormalities (dehiscence, stricture)
– Disease recurrence
▪ Complications affecting the allograft and/or native lung
– Infection
– Pleural complications (empyema, effusion)
– Pulmonary embolic disease
– Malignancy (primary lung cancer, PTLD)
▪ Complications affecting the native lung (SLT)
– Hyperinflation (emphysema)
– Pneumothorax
– Refractory infection
Non-Pulmonary Complications
▪ Cardiovascular (systemic hypertension, rhythm disturbance, thromboembolism)
▪ Renal dysfunction
▪ Cardiovascular complications (e.g., atrial fibrillation)
▪ Metabolic/endocrine
– Hyperglycemia, diabetes, obesity, dyslipidemia
– Electrolyte abnormalities, hyperammonemia
▪ Gastrointestinal
– GERD, gastroparesis, bezoar formation, biliary tract dysfunction
– bowel disorders, DIOS, colitis (neutropenic, *C. difficile* colitis)
▪ Infection
▪ Musculoskeletal (osteopenia, osteoporosis, myopathy)
▪ Hematologic (anemia, leukopenia, thrombotic microangiopathy)
▪ Neurologic
– Tremor, headache, seizure, memory loss
– CVA, blindness, coma
▪ Drug toxicity/adverse drug reactions
– Immunosuppressants (e.g., calcineurin inhibitor toxicities)
– Drug-drug interactions
▪ Malignancy (skin, primary lung, PTLD)

Abbreviations: BOS = bronchiolitis obliterans syndrome; CVA = cerebrovascular accident; DIOS = distal intestinal obstruction syndrome; GERD = gastroesophageal reflux disease; PGD =

primary graft dysfunction; PTLD = post-transplant lymphoproliferative disease; SLT = single lung transplantation.

Radiographic imaging, pulmonary function testing, and bronchoscopy are all important tools for monitoring the transplant recipient. Bronchoscopy can be done within 24-48 hrs of implantation to inspect the anastomoses and ensure that significant abnormalities such as anastomotic dehiscence have not occurred. Routine chest x-rays (CXR) are useful to gauge the extent of reperfusion injury and monitor for pleural and parenchymal changes of concern. Inhaled nitric oxide may be useful to stabilize the recipient hemodynamically and relieve pulmonary hypertension, and prophylaxis to prevent thromboembolism should be maintained until the patient is ambulatory and risk factors are no longer present. Once the patient is extubated and has adequate pain relief, spirometry can be initiated to establish a baseline and subsequently monitor physiologic function.

Fever and cough, increased lung infiltrates, and/or a fall in FEV1 can all be seen with evolving ACR or infection. However, some patients can have occult infection (e.g., CMV pneumonitis) or AR and not have overt symptoms, a change on CXR, or a decline in FEV1. Bronchoscopy with transbronchial biopsy (TBBx) and bronchoalveolar lavage (BAL) can usually retrieve diagnostic specimens and identify infection and/or rejection as a cause of clinical deterioration Patients can occasionally have signs and symptoms compatible with rejection but have a negative TBBx. In this situation, a patient may still have an alloimmune rejection response (e.g., antibody-mediated rejection); imaging and BAL can help rule out infection, and patients will usually respond to enhanced immunosuppression. Serial peripheral blood sampling with polymerase chain reaction (PCR) testing for CMV can be useful for monitoring for CMV infection/disease as well as detecting evolving CMV infection, especially for recipients whose matches that are not donor-/recipient- and, therefore, at higher risk for CMV disease.

Delayed Onset and Chronic Complications

Delayed, unexplained, persistent decline in lung allograft function has been perceived to be caused by obliteration of small airways (obliterative bronchiolitis [OB]). Because this diagnosis is difficult to make via less invasive techniques (bronchoscopy, thoracic imaging), the surrogate marker of FEV1 decline (to ≤80% of the best post-transplant FEV1 value) has been used to detect and diagnose recipients as having bronchiolitis obliterans syndrome (BOS). BOS remains the predominant cause of lung function decline, graft loss, and recipient death for lung transplant survivors beyond the first year post-transplant. However, taking a closer look at what has been perceived as BOS and attributed to chronic rejection over the past few years has revealed that different phenotypes of "BOS" exist, and the term chronic lung allograft dysfunction (CLAD) has been suggested as an overarching term for chronic lung allograft rejection that encompasses the subsets/phenotypes of (1) classical obstructive BOS, which typically lacks significant lung parenchymal changes on thoracic imaging and is characterized by obstructive physiology, and (2) restrictive allograft syndrome (RAS), which is characterized by a restrictive pattern of lung physiologic impairment accompanied by parenchymal infiltrates (both entities were historically identified simply as BOS). Recent investigations indicate that RAS has a worse prognosis than the more prevalent obstructive BOS phenotype, and responses to therapy may also differ. Risk factors associated with the development of CLAD include primary graft dysfunction, acute rejection, persistent BAL neutrophilia, lymphocytic bronchiolitis, antibody-mediated rejection, gastroesophageal reflux (GER), infections (viral, bacterial, fungal), autoimmunity, and exposure to air pollution. Additionally, it is now recognized that other factors (e.g., anastomosis dysfunction, allograft inflammatory or infectious complications, external allograft compression, primary disease recurrence, vascular obstruction) can significantly affect allograft function, may coexist with lesions of OB, and can contribute to CLAD. Another entity that has been perceived as BOS is a constrictive bronchiolitis that can improve in response to azithromycin administration such that allograft function can be restored or substantially improved and stabilized; this entity is typically characterized by BAL neutrophilia and has been termed neutrophilic reversible allograft dysfunction (NRAD). However, patients with obstructive BOS may also have a clinical response to azithromycin, and the term, azithromycin-responsive allograft dysfunction (ARAD), may be the best term for lung function decline that meets criteria for CLAD but stabilizes or improves when azithromycin is administered. Finally, some explanted allografts from recipients that met criteria for a diagnosis of BOS have been found to have relatively sparse/rare lesions of OB present on histopathology but were found to have considerable vascular remodeling and interstitial fibrosis, which supports the need for alternative terminology (e.g., CLAD and CLAD phenotypes) that can be used to replace BOS as an overarching term for chronic allograft dysfunction.

Many non-pulmonary complications must be prevented, detected in a timely fashion via appropriate monitoring, and/or treated when they occur (Table 4). Additionally, many patients already have significant problems at the time of transplantation that need to be managed appropriately and monitored (e.g., diabetes, osteoporosis, hyperlipidemia, systemic hypertension). Immunosuppressive medications must be monitored carefully, especially for effects on kidney and bone marrow function. The calcineurin inhibitors (CNI; tacrolimus or cyclosporine) affect the kidneys and can cause significant impairment of renal function (acutely if CNI levels are supratherapeutic or gradually/subacutely with sustained administration with levels that are sustained within the target range). Despite the best management, some patients may eventually develop renal failure that requires renal replacement therapy or kidney transplantation. Attention to all drugs that can affect renal function and monitoring renal function is of prime importance. Drug-drug interactions are another important cause of complications, and treating clinicians must be aware that many drugs interact with the CNIs (which are metabolized by the hepatic P-450 cytochrome system) that virtually all patients must take life-long to prevent rejection. Other complications for which monitoring is required and for which prophylactic measures or treatment is typically given include cardiovascular complications or co-morbidities (e.g., systemic hypertension, rhythm disturbances), metabolic disturbances (e.g., hyperkalemia, hyperglycemia/diabetes, hyperlipidemia), osteopenia/osteoporosis, excessive weight gain/obesity, endocrine dysfunction, gastroesophageal reflux, anemia, leukopenia, infection, and malignancy. In addition, recipients are also at risk for various metabolic disturbances, other gastrointestinal complications (e.g., altered bowel motility, biliary tract disease), neurologic complications (e.g., tremor, headache, seizure, memory loss), and malignancies such as PTLD (post-transplant lymphoproliferative disease) or other neoplasms (e.g., skin cancer, primary lung cancer).

Post-Transplant Surveillance

In addition to assessing allograft status and pulmonary physiology, routine surveillance to detect and manage post-transplant medical complications in the outpatient setting should include a comprehensive patient interview with a complete medication history to ensure compliance with treatment regimens, vital signs (especially to detect systemic hypertension), a careful physical examination, and peripheral blood testing as appropriate (e.g., calcineurin inhibitor [CNI] and mammalian target of rapamycin (mTOR) inhibitor levels, complete blood count, electrolytes, renal function). Intermittent monitoring of bone marrow function via complete blood counts with differential cell count performed at regular intervals will allow detection of bone marrow suppression (e.g., anemia, leukopenia, thrombocytopenia) that may occur as a consequence of chronic immunosuppressive therapy.

The routine use of surveillance bronchoscopy (SB) for monitoring lung allograft function is somewhat controversial, and only 2/3 of transplant centers in the US perform routine surveillance bronchoscopy. Bronchoscopy can detect occult infection or AR when done for surveillance purposes in patients who appear to be stable and lack radiographic or physiologic signs of allograft dysfunction, especially during the first 6 months post-transplant. However, the benefits of detecting lower grades of ACR and treating it are not clear (e.g., better survival, lower risk of developing CLAD/BOS). Although even minimal (A1) ACR has been associated with increased risk for developing chronic rejection and CLAD, no clear benefit has been shown for SB detection of ACR and intensification of immunosuppressive therapy to suppress ACR with the hope of diminishing the risk of subsequently developing CLAD. Another limitation of SB is the very limited ability to diagnose the presence of OB as a correlate of chronic rejection, necessitating use of the surrogate marker of lung function (FEV1) for detecting the onset of CLAD/BOS and gauging the severity of chronic allograft dysfunction. Lastly, there is a small but not insignificant risk of complications with SB (hemorrhage, pneumothorax, lower tract infection), and safety protocols should be in place to minimize the risk of these complications.

Diagnosing acute and chronic allograft rejection can be very challenging for young children with CF. Children under 4 years of age typically have difficulty performing spirometry, and alternative techniques to measure lung function or imaging techniques (e.g., high-resolution computed tomography with inspiratory and expiratory views, ventilation-perfusion scans) may be used as alternative methods to detect allograft dysfunction. Because bronchoscopy with transbronchial biopsies are difficult to perform in young children, surgical lung biopsy may be needed to establish or confirm suspected BOS/CLAD.

OUTCOMES

Compared to other types of solid organ transplant, long-term survival for lung or heart-lung transplant recipients is significantly worse than that for single organ heart, kidney, or liver recipients but is comparable or exceeds that for lung recipients with other indications for transplant (Table 5). However, when compared to other indications for lung transplantation (such as IPF or COPD), post-transplant survival for adult patients with CF is not worse despite the challenges of ongoing risk for infection and extrapulmonary comorbidities. Data from the international registry maintained by the International Society for Heart and Lung Transplantation indicated a median survival of 8.3 years for patients with CF for the most recent era, and Kaplan-Meier estimated survival for 100 consecutive patients with CF transplanted at our own institution at 10 years post-transplant is 58%. However, long-term complications for which all lung transplant recipients are at risk regardless of transplant indication (systemic hypertension, dyslipidemia, impaired kidney function, CLAD) will eventually appear in most lung recipients with CF.

Table 5. 1- and 3-Year Survival for Solid Organ Transplantation in the United States[*]

Organ	1-Year Graft Survival	3-Year Graft Survival
Lung (adults; all indications)	86.5% (N = 4,575) (7/1/2012-12/31/2014)[**]	63.7% (N = 4,333) (1/10/2010-6/30/2012)[**]
Lung (adults; CF as indication)	85.2% (N = 461) (1997-2004)[**]	64.1% (N = 419) (1997-2004)[**]
Lung (adults; COPD as indication)	86.2% (N = 1,049) (1997-2004)[**]	65.1% (N = 1,051) (1997-2004)[**]
Lung (adults; IPF as indication)	79.0% (N = 544) (1997-2004)[**]	55.6% (N = 351) (1997-2004)[**]
Lung (pediatric; all indications)	86.4% (N = 120) (1997-2004)[**]	61.1% (N = 111) (1997-2004)[**]
Heart-Lung	84.1% (N = 44) (7/1/2012-12/31/2014)[**]	57.8% (N = 79) (1/10/2010-6/30/2012)[**]
Heart	90.3% (N = 5,096) (7/1/2012-12/31/2014)[**]	83.5% (N = 4,735) (1/10/2010-6/30/2012)[**]
Kidney (deceased donor)	93.6% (N = 13,485) (7/1/2012-12/31/2014)[**]	84.7% (N = 24,728) (1/10/2010-6/30/2012)[**]
Kidney (living donor)	97.5% (N = 13,485) (7/1/2012-12/31/2014)[**]	91.9% (N = 14,081) (1/10/2010-6/30/2012)[**]
Liver (deceased donor)	88.8% (N = 13,068) (7/1/2012-12/31/2014)[**]	79.2% (N = 12,801) (1/10/2010-6/30/2012)[**]

Organ	1-Year Graft Survival	3-Year Graft Survival
Liver (living donor)	84.1% (N = 544) (7/1/2012-12/31/2014)**	Not available
Intestine	68.3% (N = 169) (7/1/2012-12/31/2014)**	54.8% (N = 175) (1/10/2010-6/30/2012)**

* Data for National Graft Survival from Scientific Registry of Transplant Recipients (www.srtr.org/csr/current/centers/default.aspx – released July 2012).

** Time window when transplants were performed.

Kaplan-Meier Survival Rates.

Abbreviations: CF – cystic fibrosis; COPD = chronic obstructive pulmonary disease; IPF = idiopathic pulmonary fibrosis.

CF-related diabetes (CFRD), osteopenia/osteoporosis, GERD, and hepatobiliary tract dysfunction are already present at the time of transplantation for many patients, and these can worsen after transplant or appear *de novo* in recipients who lacked such complications pre-transplant. Over one third of CF lung recipients will develop new-onset CFRD following transplant. Although a significant impact on post-transplant outcomes has not been demonstrated for CFRD per se, but aggressive management is needed both before and after lung transplant. Osteoporosis is common in patients pre-transplant, and thoracic compression fractures with poorly controlled pain is a situation that is considered a contraindication to lung transplant by most centers; however, aggressive therapy with bisphosphonates combined with vitamin D and calcium supplementation can maintain or even improve bone mineral density in adults with CF. Patients with evidence of hepatic cirrhosis are at increased risk for post-transplant complications, but isolated lung transplant can usually be performed safely at large volume centers if liver disease is mild.

Another significant challenge is persistent bacterial colonization/infection in paranasal sinuses and proximal native airways that can be trans-located into the lung allografts and cause allograft infection. The sinuses serve as reservoirs of infection, and there is high concordance of bacterial isolates from paranasal sinus aspirates with bacteria identified in BAL specimens obtained at bronchoscopy. Endoscopic sinus surgery plus subsequent nasal rinsing can diminish both sinus and lower respiratory tract bacterial colonization and may have an impact on both freedom from CLAD and survival.

Recipients with CF are also at risk for numerous gastrointestinal complications that include new onset or worsened GERD, gastric bezoar formation that can impair bioavailability of orally administered immunosuppressive drugs, intestinal dysmotility that may lead to distal intestinal obstruction syndrome (DIOS), *Clostridium difficile* colitis, or neoplasia (especially colon cancer). Patients with CF are at increased risk for gastrointestinal malignancy (especially colon cancer) even at young ages and outside of the setting of having received a solid organ transplant; when and how frequently screening to detect and remove colonic neoplasms (e.g., pre-neoplastic polyps) should occur is an issue that remains unclear.

CONCLUSION

Patients with CF present many unique challenges to care providers both before and after lung transplantation. However, patients with CF who undergo lung transplantation report improved quality of life with improved physical and social functioning, better energy levels, improved sleep quality, and a reduced treatment burden. Although lung transplantation for young children may be controversial in terms of survival outcomes, a survival benefit for adult patients at high risk of short-term mortality, which is generally reflected by a high LAS value, is not considered controversial, and lung transplantation is an appropriate option for patients with CF who are at high risk for short-term mortality. However, major challenges to optimal post-transplant outcomes include early surgical complications due to technical issues, primary graft dysfunction leading to allograft failure, early and late infectious complications, and BOS/CLAD.

New approaches that are needed to optimize recipient and allograft survival following transplantation include (1) identifying immunosuppressive regimens that optimally prevent post-transplant allograft rejection yet minimize the risk of opportunistic infection, (2) prophylactic antimicrobial therapies to prevent opportunistic infections, and, most importantly, (3) an improved understanding of CLAD and allograft rejection that will lead to advances that prevent the development of CLAD and its subsets of obstructive BOS or RAS (as well as therapies that can arrest progressive loss of allograft function should CLAD develop). Lastly, appropriate palliative measures need to be incorporated into post-transplant management protocols to relieve symptoms when recipients develop refractory loss of allograft function due to the appearance of advanced and progressive CLAD, and retransplantation can be considered for patients who develop severe allograft dysfunction due to CLAD.

REFERENCES

[1] Weill D, Benden C, Corris PA, A consensus document for the selection of lung transplant candidates: 2014-an update from the Pulmonary Transplantation Council of the International Society for Heart and Lung Transplantation. *J Heart Lung Transplant.* 2015 Jan;34(1):1-15.

[2] *Lung Transplantation.* Eds. Vigneswaran WT, Garrity ER Jr. Informa Healthcare Ltd. New York, 2010.

[3] Spahr JE, Love RB, Francois M, Radford K, Meyer KC. Lung transplantation for cystic fibrosis: current concepts and one center's experience. *J Cyst Fibros.* 2007 Sep;6(5):334-50.

[4] Spahr J, Meyer K. Lung transplantation. In: *Primer on Transplantation* (3rd Edition). Ed. Hricik D, American Society of Transplantation; Wiley-Blackwell, Oxford, UK, 2011, pp. 205-237.

[5] Meyer KC, Raghu G, Verleden GM, Corris PA, Aurora P, Wilson KC, Brozek J, Glanville AR; ISHLT/ATS/ERS BOS Task Force Committee. An international ISHLT/ATS/ERS clinical practice guideline: diagnosis and management of bronchiolitis obliterans syndrome. *Eur Respir J* 2014 Dec;44(6):1479-503.

[6] Bronchiolitis Obliterans Syndrome. Editors: Meyer KC, Glanville A; Springer; Humana Press, New York, 2013 (Respiratory Medicine; Series Editor Sharon Rounds).

[7] Meyer KC. Lung transplantation: chronic complications and management. In: *Lung Transplantation*, Eds. Vigneswaran WT and Garrity ER. Informa Healthcare Ltd, New York, 2010; pages 357-374.

[8] Meyer KC. Medical Complications of the Lung Transplant Patient. In: *Lung Transplantation: Principles and Practice.* Eds. Vigneswaran W, Garrity E, Odell J. CRC Press 2015; pages 371-383.

[9] Dasenbrook E, Merlo C. Cystic fibrosis and bronchiectasis. In: *Lung Transplantation*, Eds. Vigneswaran WT and Garrity ER. Informa Healthcare Ltd, New York, 2010; pages 58-64.

[10] Hayes D Jr, Meyer KC. Lung transplantation for advanced bronchiectasis. *Semin Respir Crit Care Med* 2010;31;123-138.

[11] *Lung Transplantation: Principles and Practice.* Eds. Vigneswaran WT, Garrity ER Jr, Odell JA. CRC Press, Taylor and Francis; 2016.

[12] Dark JH. *Lung transplantation for cystic fibrosis and bronchiectasis.* CRC Press, Taylor and Francis; 2016; pages 203-210.

[13] Blatter J, Sweet S. Lung transplantation in cystic fibrosis: trends and controversies. *Pediatr Allergy Immunol Pulmonol.* 2015 Dec. 1;28(4): 237-243.

[14] Yusen RD, Edwards LB, Kucheryavaya AY, Benden C, Dipchand AI, Dobbels F, Goldfarb SB, Levvey BJ, Lund LH, Meiser B, Stehlik J; International Society for Heart and Lung Transplantation. The registry of the International Society for Heart and Lung Transplantation: thirty-first adult lung and heart-lung transplant report-2014; focus theme: retransplantation. *J Heart Lung Transplant.* 2014 Oct;33(10):1009-24.

In: Cystic and Idiopathic Pulmonary Fibrosis ISBN: 978-1-63485-508-2
Editor: Lorenzo Robertson

Chapter 4

NEW CYSTIC FIBROSIS THERAPY

Sabrine Oueslati*

Biochemistry Laboratory, Children's Hospital; Research laboratory "Haemoglobinopathies and Cystic fibrosis, LR00SP03", Tunis, Tunisia

ABSTRACT

Cystic fibrosis (CF) is a lethal monogenic disease with an early mortality and morbidity. It is caused by mutations in the gene encoding the cystic fibrosis transmembrane conductance regulator (CFTR) that *engenders* thick, sticky mucus to form in the lungs, pancreas, and other organs. Survival and quality of life have improved, through better management of nutrition and, respiratory infections, rather than through interventions that target the basic defect. In fact, *therapy* for CF has progressed during the past several decades. Withal, with more than 2000 mutations that can produce a faulty CFTR, the management of CF remains a challenge. Several innovative drugs recently approved by the Food and Drug Administration, termed genetic modulators, target the underlying disease by modulating the CFTR defect.

Nowadays, many *innovations have concerned the daily treatment of CF*, focus on inhaled and oral medications and optimized nutrition, such as the development of drugs with "intelligent nebulisers" and dry-powder inhalers becoming commonplace. These developments have occurred in conjunction with development of a wider variety of therapeutic strategies. In fact, new therapeutic strategies have been developed to target various

* sabrineoueslati@yahoo.fr.

aspects of the physiological *waterfall in* CF. The development of Oral agents such as ivacaftor, which work for selected genotypes to directly potentiate the cystic fibrosis transmembrane conductance regulator (CFTR) protein and *lumacaftor* to correct intracellular processing of CFTR offer huge potential to target the underlying defects in specific CFTR mutations and alter the disease process, and could be life-changing. The vast majority of efforts over the last 20 years have focused on developing a gene therapy for CF lung disease largely due to the urgent need for more effective treatments and the noninvasive accessibility of the lung also the gene therapy approach is potential use in all mutation classes.

Over the past few decades, remarkable improvements have been made in clinical outcomes for CF patients including better nutritional status, new target and gene therapy. Many drug have also been developed to improve the quality of life of patients.

INTRODUCTION

Cystic fibrosis (CF) is one of the most common autosomal recessive disorders in the Caucasian population. The CF transmembrane conductance regulator (*CFTR*) gene responsible for this disease consists of 27 exons, spanning approximately 250 kb located on the long arm of chromosome 7 at position 7q31.2 (Welsh MJ et al., 2013) and encodes a 1480 amino acid: the cystic fibrosis transmembrane conductance regulator (CFTR) protein located in the apical membrane of epithelial cells (Collins FS, 1992). CFTR protein has several functions including cAMPdependent chloride and bicarbonate secretion and regulation of epithelial sodium channels (ENaCs). The dysfunction of this protein affect multiple organs, including the intestine, sweat glands, pancreas and the reproductive system, but lung disease represent the major cause of morbidity and early mortality in cystic fibrosis patients. It is estimated that over 90% of deaths due to CF are attributable to lung disease, the culmination of early and persistent infections that lead to structural changes over time, progressive airway obstruction and ultimately respiratory failure (Flume, 2009). Over the past few decades, survival and quality of life have been improved, through better management of nutrition and, respiratory infections, rather than through interventions that target the basic defect. In fact, since the discovery of *CFTR* gene in 1989, many progresses in CF *therapy* was obtained.

EVOLUTION OF CF THERAPY

Since the discovery of the disease, the treatment is just intended to alleviate the symptoms of CF patients. Nowadays, remarkable improvements have been made in clinical research, including better nutritional status (Stephenson et al., 2013), progressive reductions in the annual rate of decline of lung function (Que et al., 2006) and steady improvements in expected survival (Dodge et al., 2007).

NUTRITIONAL MANAGEMENT

More than 85% of patients are pancreatic insufficient at birth and others gradually lose function over time. Improving the nutritional status of CF patients is ensured by the administration of pancreatic enzymes preparation. Indeed, the exocrine pancreas plays a key role in the digestive function through the secretion of pancreatic juice, consisting of numerous enzymes, and of aqueous solution rich in sodium bicarbonate (Fiker et al., 2011). In CF patients, the pathological changes in the pancreas of duct obstruction and destruction of acinar cells occur as a result of abnormalities of the CFTR protein. This leads to abnormal transmembrane fluid and electrolyte movement. A deficiency of pancreatic bicarbonate reduces duodenal pH, inactivating pancreatic enzymes and precipitating bile salts (Gilbert et al., 1988; Geus et al., 1999). There is increased fecal loss of bile salts (Walters et Littlewood, 1998) and a relative increase in glycine-conjugated and a decrease in taurine-conjugated bile salts (Roy et al., 1977). Glycine-conjugated bile salts are less effective at lipid solubilization. Intestinal mucosal ion transport abnormalities affecting both water and electrolyte transport appear to be related to the basic CFTR defect (Sinaasappel, 1992). Impaired mucosal uptake and transport of long-chain fatty acids may occur (Kalivianakis et al., 1999; Laiho et al., 2004). There is also an altered motility, with an increased small bowel transit time (Littlewood et al., 2006).

Pancreatic insufficiency (PI) leads to impaired digestion and the fat soluble vitamins A, D, E and K (Dodge, 2006). The presence in CF patient of fat in the stools (steatorrhoea) leading to a failure to gain weight accompanied by a malnutrition, resulting from poor absorption of vitamins. That is why, as soon as the diagnosis of CF is made the pancreatic enzyme replacement therapy (PERT) is routinely administered to the patients to prevent the symptoms of fat malabsorption including frequent pale, oily and offensive stools, abdominal pain, poor growth and deficiencies of fat soluble vitamins and essential fatty acids (Wolfe et Morton, 2006). Orally administered pancreatic enzymes have been available since at least the 19th century, when many formulations were available as digestive aids. At that time it was known that orally administered enzymes were destroyed in gastric juice and that they were most effective when given in alkaline media (Trang et al., 2014).

Pancreatic enzyme replacement therapy varies among patients depending on the type of food being eaten, the degree of malabsorption, age of patient, the acidity in the gut, the gastrointestinal transit time…There are a various of enzyme preparations available (Littlewood *et al.*, 2006). Usully, they are given to CF patients orally 10 to 20 minutes before meals and snacks, either as tablets, enteric coated or non enteric coated capsules (for those individuals able to swallow a capsule) or as granules (for infants and young children) (Fiker et al., 2011).

In terms of lung disease, removal of mucus and secretions with chest physiotherapy and the development of more advanced lung clearance devices and techniques. Nowadays, many innovations have concerned the daily treatment of CF, focus on inhaled and oral medications and airway clearance, such as the development of drugs with "intelligent nebulisers" and dry-powder inhalers. In fact, Inhaled therapies offer targeted drug delivery and are relatively simple, efficient and quick to take. The inhaled medications are released in a targeted way in the airways of CF patients and coupled with limited systemic toxicity (Agent P et Parrott H, 2015). This therapy aims to preserve lung function as well as reducing exacerbation risk, plays a key role in mitigating the risks associated with lung infections in CF (Fiel, 2014). International guidelines recommend long-term inhaled antibiotics for patients with CF and chronic P. aeruginosa infection (Mogayzel et al., 2013; Smyth et al., 2014). Nebulised carbenicillin and gentamycin were first used (Hodson et al., 1981). recent advances have focused on dry-powder developments, with formulations currently available for tobramycin (TOBI Podhaler; Novartis Pharmaceuticals, East Hanover, NJ, USA) and colistin (Colobreathe; Forest Laboratories, Dartford, UK) (Agent et Parrott, 2015). A number of other inhaled antibiotics are currently being evaluated in clinical studies. The progress in inhalator therapy offer simple, fast and convenient delivery of inhaled antibiotics, while delivering similar efficacy to nebulised formulations. In addition, dry-powder inhalers require minimal cleaning compared with a nebuliser system, which is also time consuming and often not performed to recommended manufacturer's guidance (Agent et Parrott, 2015).

These developments have occurred in conjunction with the emergence of a wider variety of therapeutic strategies. In fact, new therapeutic strategies have been developed to target various aspects of the physiological waterfall in CF caused by different mutations of *CFTR* gene. To date, more than 2,000 mutations of the *CFTR* gene have been identified (http://www.genet.sickkids.on.ca/StatisticsPage.html). The distribution of CFTR mutations varies depending to the ethnicity of patients (Cuppens and Cassiman, 2004). Additional, approximately only 20 mutations have a frequency >0.1% (Roganet al., 2011). In fact, notwithstanding the common F508del variant, only four CFTR mutations have a frequency 0.1%: G551D, W1282X, G542X and N1303K, having a worldwide prevalence of around 1–3% each (Roganet al., 2011; Clancy and Jain, 2012). F508del is the most common mutation with an allelic frequency of around 90% worldwide (cystic fibrosis genetic analysis consortium, 1990; Amaral MD and Kunzelmann K, 2007). In order to understand the new CFTR treatments designed to correct the basic CFTR defect, the mechanisms of CFTR dysfunction need to be understood *(Boyle et De Boeck, 2013). CFTR* mutations are divided into six classes based on the mechanisms that are affected: CFTR synthesis, trafficking or function (Zielenski and Tsui, 1995; Haardt et al., 1999). For class I mutations, like G542X and W1282X mutation, there is a premature termination of the CFTR mRNA translation caused by a nucleotide substitution introducingan in-frame premature termination codon (PTC) – UAA, UAG or UGA–, frame-shifting insertions or deletions, mutations at the invariant dinucleotide splice junctions, or introduction of a PTC, resulting in complete skipping of an out of frame exon, (4) a complete or partial deletion of the CFTR gene or (5)a rearrangement in the gene altering the exon sequence. Mutations that generate PTCs can reduce the level of mRNA via non-sense-mediated decay (NMD), which degrades the abnormal PTC-containing mRNA (Maquat, 1995; Fanen et al., 2014). The most common mutation F508del and the N1303K mutation belong to class II mutations and result in defects in protein processing. In this class, the misfolded protein is retained in the endoplasmic reticulum (ER), retro-translocated to the cytoplasm, where it is degraded by the ubiquitin/proteasome pathway (Jensen et al., 1995; Ward et al., 1995). The third class contain mutations frequently located in the ATP bindingd omains (NBD1 and NBD2) and are referred to as gating mutations. They are missense mutations producing a protein efficiently inserted in the membrane at normal levels, but resistant to activation by protein kinase A. The G551D mutation is an example of this class. Class IV mutations result in protein reaching the plasma membrane, but it has altered channel properties that results in defective protein conduction. The missense mutations located in these regions producea protein efficiently inserted in the membrane, which retains acAMP-dependent Cl−channel activity, but with a reduced chan-nel conductance. Alleles in this class are typically associated witha milder form of the disease (Fanen et al., 2014). The R117H and R347P mutations are examples of class IV mutations. Class V mutations result in reduced amounts of RNA necessary for normal CFTR production. In fact, most of the class V mutations reduce the total amount of CFTR protein by affecting pre-mRNA splicing. These splice site mutations can induce complete or partial exclusion of an exon. In the latter case, production of normal mRNA is maintained, but in lower quantity. When the skipped exon is in phase, the transcript will produce an incomplete non-functional channel. On the other hand, when the skipped exon is out of phase, a PTC will rapidly appear and the transcript will be degraded by the NMD (non sense mediated mRNA decay) pathway (Fanen et al., 2014). The VI class of mutations are now combined with class V, as mutations leading to reduce functional CFTR protein (Welsh et al., 2001). The landscape of CF therapeutics changed dramatically with the development of target therapy 'mutation-specific treatment'. These therapies have been driven by the concepts of precision and stratified medicine, whereby molecular biomarkers can be used to select specific approaches for individuals or groups of individuals, respectively, enabling the production of highly effective and precise treatments (Collins et Varmus, 2015).

Some of the advantages of targeted therapies include the ability to identify treatment responders, tailor treatment to an individual's genetic profile, and avoid unwanted side effects (Hall, 2013). This approach is in direct contrast to most drugs currently used in medical practice, which are used to treat large populations with the same broad disease label but with marked heterogeneity in response to treatment (Brodlie et al., 2015).

The developement of Ivacaftor new treatment for CF has made a huge turning point in the treatment of cystic fibrosis. In fact, Ivacaftor (previously called VX-770) is a small drug molecule *N*-(2,4-Di-*tert*-butyl-5-hydroxyphenyl)-4-oxo-1,4-dihydroquinoline-3-carboxamide ($C_{24}H_{28}N_2O_3$) (Figure 1). Ivacaftor was approved by the Food and Drug Administration in 2012 and have 'KALYDECO' as a commercial name. It was licensed in the United States and Europe for use in patients with CF aged six years and over who carry at least one copy of the class III mutation, Gly551Asp. Ivacaftor is available as a light blue capsule shaped, film coated tablet for oral administration containing 150 mg of ivacafor as oral granules containing 50 or

75 mg of ivacaftor. The oral granules are indicated for 2-5 year olds and are administered in liquid or soft foods within 1 hour of mixing.

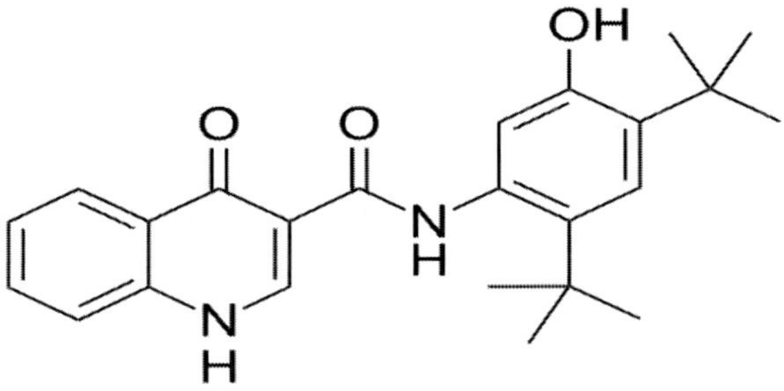

Figure 1. Chemical structure of ivacaftor.

Ivacaftor is an orally bioavailable agent that is designed to increase the time that activated CFTR channels at the cell surface remain open (a "potentiator") (Ramsey et al., 2011). It was identified via high-throughput screening involving a library of nearly 230,000 potential therapeutic compounds (Ledford, 2012). Based on in vitro and pharmacologic studies and safety profiles, this drug was demonstrated as a potentiator of CFTR function in cell culture with respiratory epithelial cells that carried a single Gly551Asp (G551D) mutation (Van Goor., 2009). The G551D mutation, belongs to the III classe, is a missense mutation in which the amino acid glycine is substituted for aspartate at position 551 in the nucleotide-binding domain-1 of the gene. *This mutation leads to* a normal quantity of protein available in the plasma membrane but with reduced open probability of the channel, thus resulting in severely impaired CFTR function.

Clinical Trials of Ivacaftor in Patients with the Gly551Asp CFTR Mutation

Ivacaftor was identified by screening over of 228,000 small-molecule compounds using high throughput screening with a cell-based fluorescence membrane potential assay designed to identify CFTR potentiators (Van Goor et al., 2009). In vitro studies, developed on both recombinant cell lines and primary cultures of human bronchial epithelial cells, have demonstrated that ivacaftor increases chloride transport by increasing the probability of the CFTR channel being open, and increases apical fluid height and ciliary beat frequency (Van Goor et al., 2009; O'Reilly et Elphick, 2013). Further studies elaborated on the mechanism of action of ivacaftor at the CFTR channel have shown that the drug opens the defective channel gate of mutant CFTR in a phosphorylation dependent but ATP independent manner (Eckford et al., 2012).

A phase II double-blinded placebo-controlled trial was performed. Measures of CFTR function included nasal potential difference (as a marker of chloride conductance in the nasal epithelium) and sweat chloride concentration (as a readout of chloride reabsorption by CFTR in the sweat duct). Lung function was measured in terms of percentage of predicted FEV_1. Quality of life was assessed using the revised Cystic Fibrosis Questionnaire (CFQ-R). Patients aged 18≥ years with at least one Gly551Asp allele and a predicted FEV_1 of at least 40% were included in the study. The first stage of the study had a crossover design in which patients were randomly assigned to receive varying doses of ivacaftor (25 mg, 75 mg, 150 mg or placebo) every 12 hours over two 14-day periods with a washout time between these periods. The second stage was a parallel study, which involved new patients who were randomly assigned to receive varying doses of ivacaftor (150 mg, 250 mg or placebo) every 12 hours over 28 consecutive days (Accurso et al., 2010). They found a partial improvement in nasal potential difference and significant improvements in sweat chloride concentrations in individuals who received ivacaftor. The median reduction in sweat chloride levels after 28 days in the 150 mg ivacaftor group was −59.5 mmol/L versus a gain of 5 mmol/L in the placebo group. Interestingly, although still significant, the reduction in sweat chloride levels was smaller in those who received 250 mg than in those who received 150 mg of the drug. There were no significant improvements in FEV_1 in patients who received ivacaftor versus placebo. However, there were significant within-subject improvements in FEV_1 from baseline with the 75 mg and 150 mg doses. Health-related quality of life was better with ivacaftor, but the changes were not significant. Although this study clearly demonstrated the benefits of ivacaftor in patients with cystic fibrosis, it was limited by its small sample size, which may have contributed towards the lack of significance found with some outcome measures (Accurso et al., 2010).

To determine safety and efficacy of ivafactor in CF patients carried at least the Gly551Asp mutation in one allele has been assessed in two larger phase III double-blinded randomized controlled trials. *Patients included in these studies* were clinically stable and have 12 years of age or older (n= 161) in the first study (STRIVE study) (Ramsey et al., 2011) and the second one (ENVISION study) included 52 children aged between 6 and 12 years (Davies et al., 2013). The primary efficacy endpoint in both studies was the mean absolute change from baseline in forced expiratory volume in one second (FEV_1) percent predicted at 24 weeks from baseline. Patients in both trials were randomized in a 1:1 ratio to receive either 150 mg of ivacaftor or placebo orally every 12 hours for 48 weeks, in addition to their usual CF therapies prescribed prestudy (Ramsey et al., 2011; Davies et al., 2013). In the adult and adolescent group, 70% of trial participants were on regular dornase alfa and 50% were on nebulized tobramycin (Ramsey et al., 2011). Use of inhaled hypertonic saline was not permitted because it does not have regulatory approval in the United States as a therapy for CF (Ramsey et al., 2011). Ivacaftor was given with foods containing fat because this increases the exposure by 2 to 4 fold (Davies et al., 2013). Ivacaftor therapy resulted in a significant improvement in lung function (10.6% absolute difference in FEV1), a significant reduction in pulmonary exacerbations and a significant increase in weight (Ramsey et al., 2011). The substantial effects on lung function were mirrored in a study of ivacaftor therapy in a paediatric Population (Davies et al., 2013). In both studies, ivacaftor therapy significantly reduced sweat chloride levels, providing evidence of effect on the CFTR protein channel and, in many patients, returned sweat chloride levels to below the diagnostic threshold for CF (Ramsey et al., 2011; Davies et al., 2013). Interestingly, in the trials, decreases in sweat chloride did not correlate with improvement in FEV_1 in those treated with ivacaftor (Durmowicz et al., 2013). The effects of ivacaftor have also been studied in patients with severe impairment of lung function with an FEV_1 percent predicted to be $\leq 40\%$ (Barry et al., 2014). Significant improvements in lung function, number of days of intravenous antibiotic therapy, weight and body mass index (BMI) were found among patients after treatment in a retrospective case–control study (Barry et al., 2014).

Use of ivacaftor in patients with severe hepatic dysfunction (Child-Pugh class C) is cautioned; if used, the dose should be reduced to 150 mg daily or less frequently. In patients with moderate impairment (Child-Pugh class B), the dose should be reduced to 150 mg daily (Product information. Kalydeco, 2012). No dosage modifications are recommended for patients with renal impairment but caution should be used in patients with end stage renal disease or creatinine clearance less than or equal to 30 mL/min. Drug interaction monitoring is important for ivacaftor since it is a CYP3A substrate and a weak inhibitor of CYP3A, P-glycoprotein, CYP2C8, and CYP2C9 (Product information. Kalydeco, 2012). Avoiding grapefruit juice and Seville oranges is also recommended during ivacaftor therapy.hepatic.

CLINICAL TRIALS OF IVACAFTOR IN PATIENTS WITH CFTR MUTATION OTHER THAN G551D

The success of ivacaftor therapy in patients carrying the G551D mutation has led to its study in patients who carry other class III mutations. *In vitro* there are evidence that ivacaftor potentiates the CFTR function in other class III *CFTR* mutations (Van Goor et al., 2009; Yu et al., 2012). In fact, in a panel of Fischer rat thyroid (FRT) cells expressing G551D, G178R, G551S, G970R, G1244E, S1255P, and G1349, the study of Yu et al. in 2012 confirmed that all these mutant CFTR forms shared similar in vitro functional characteristics that were consistent with a defect in channel gating. *Furthermore,* 3 additional mutations, S549N, S549R, and S1251N *also display characteristics* consistent with gating defects. These characteristics included the delivery of CFTR to the cell surface, a low (<5%) CFTR channel open probability, and minimal (<10% normal CFTR) baseline levels of chloride transport (Yu et al., 2012). Ivacaftor addition caused a >10 fold increase in CFTR-mediated chloride transport in FRT cells. For all patients the level of chloride transport achieved in the presence of ivacaftor was>10% of normal CFTR, which exceeds the level of chloride transport associated with lower sweat chloride levels and a mild CF phenotype (Davis et al., 1996). In 2014, a study elaborated by De Boeck et al. *has showed the positive impact of ivacaftor in CF patients'* non-G551D gating mutation. This study included patients who were ≥6 -years-old and carried one of the following CFTR mutations on ≥1 allele were eligible for inclusion: G178R, S549N, S549R, G551S, G970R, G1244E, S1251N, S1255P,or G1349D.

This trial contained two parts. In Part 1, ligible patients were randomized 1:1 to 1 of 2 treatment sequences: 20 with ivacaftor 150 mg q12h for 8 weeks followed by placebo q12h for 8 weeks (sequence 1, ivacaftor→placebo) or 19 with placebo q12h for 8 weeks followed by ivacaftor 150 mg q12h for 8 weeks (sequence 2, placebo→ivacaftor). The primary outcome measure was the absolute change from baseline in percent predicted FEV1through 8 weeks of ivacaftor treatment. Secondary outcome measures included the absolute change from baseline in BMI at 8 weeks of treatment; sweat chloride through 8 weeks of treatment and respiratory domain score of the Cystic Fibrosis Questionnaire-Revised (CFQ-R) through 8 weeks of treatment. In second part, all patients received ivacaftor 150 mg q12h for 16 weeks. Thus, patients randomized to treatment sequence 1(ivacaftor→placebo) had a maximum of 16 weeks of continuous ivacaftor treatment; patients randomized to treatment sequence 2 had a maximum of 24 weeks of continuous ivacaftor treatment (De Boeck et al., 2014).

Patients receiving ivacaftor demonstrated a significant improvement in absolute percent predicted FEV_1 (7.5 percentage points) through 8 weeks of treatment, whereas FEV_1declined in patients receiving placebo (−3.2 percentage points). BMI at week 8 was greater during treatment with ivacaftor (0.7 kg/m^2)compared with placebo (0.02 kg/m^2), a significant decline in sweat chloride in patients with ivacaftor treatment was observed and the CFQ-R respiratory domain score through week 8 was significantly greater in patients treated with ivacaftor (8.9 points) compared with patients receiving placebo. After the 16 week extension, FEV_1 through week 24 of ivacaftor treatment was 13.5 percentage points, BMI at week 24 was 1.3 kg/m^2 and the mean absolute change from baseline in sweat chloride through week 24 was 59.2 mmol/L. Ivacaftor safety in patients with mutation other than the G551D was evaluated by the analysis of ifections, respiratory disorders, and gastrointestinal disorder in the two parts of the study. In this study, efficacy could not be established in people with the *G970R* mutation. KALYDECO is not indicated for people with CF who have the *G970R* mutation. In conclusion treatment with ivacaftor was generally well tolerated. This study was demonstrated that patients with CF who have selected non G551D gating mutations (excepted *G970R* mutation) show clinical and pharmacodynamic improvements in response to treatment with ivacaftor that are similar to the benefits observed in patients with CF who have a G551D gating mutation (De Boeck et al., 2014).

KALYDECO (150mg, q12h) was approved by the U.S. Food and Drug Administration in February 2014 for use in people with CF ages 6 and older who have the following additional CFTR mutations: G178R, S549N, S549R, G551S, G1244E, S1251N, S1255P and G1349D. Likewise, the U.S. Food and Drug Administration approved, in Decembre 2014, the use of Kalydeco (ivacaftor) in people with cystic fibrosis (CF) ages 6 and older who have the R117H mutation. This approval is based on data from a Phase 3 study of ivacaftor that enrolled 69 people with CF who had the R117H mutation. In fact this study has shown a significant reductions in sweat chloride concentration with ivacaftor treatment. A non significant 2.1% increase in the mean absolute change from baseline in percent predicted FEV_1 ($P = 0.2$) was observed, but in a subgroup analysis of patients at least 18 years old found a statistically significant 5% difference in the mean absolute change from baseline in percent predicted FEV_1 ($P = 0.01$) adult patients demonstrated improvements in lung function (FEV_1) and CFQ-R (Vertex Pharmaceuticals, 2013).

TARGETED THERAPIES FOR PATIENTS WITH PHE508DEL CFTR MUTATION

F508del mutation is the most common mutation in CF, corresponding to the deletion of three base pairs between nucleotides 1519 to 1524 and causing a deletion of Phenylalanine in position 508 of the CFTR protein. This deletion is located in the first nucleotide-binding domain. F508del mutation affecting approximately 90% of CF patients (Park et al., 2016). The F508del mutation causes protein misfolding that results in degradation in the endoplasmic reticulum (Thomas et al., 1992). Thus, only a small amount of CFTR protein is trafficked to the cell surface (Denning et al., 1992). Once at the cell surface, the small amount of F508del CFTR that is present demonstrates defective gating and increased turnover (Kuk et Taylor-Cousar, 2015). Several early generation correctors of F508del trafficking, small molecules such as corr 4a, VRT-325 and VRT-532 (Van Goor et al., 2006), were not suitable for clinical testing due to low oral bioavailability or anticipated toxicity (Bosch et De Boeck, 2015). Correcting the function of F508del represents a challenge, that is why, several studies have been conducted in order to find an appropriate targeted therapy for this mutation (Cai et al., 2011). The most important was the ivacaftor. In fact, in vitro work in in human bronchial epithelial human epithelial cells (HBEC) homozygous for the F508del showed that ivacaftor improved CFTR mediated chloride secretion to approximately 10% of non-CF HBEC (Van Goor et al., 2009). A phase II study was performed in 140 CF patients aged ≥12 years and homozygous for the F508del mutation. Ptients was received in blinded fashion ivacaftor or placebo for 16 weeks, which was followed by an open-label extension period for patients who had demonstrated a pre-specified clinical response in the first part of the study. In fact, in the randomized part, there was a change in percentage predicted FEV1, with safety also assessed, along with sweat chloride concentration, weight and CFQ-R scores (Flume et al., 2012). There was no significant difference in predicted FEV1 in the two studied groups (Ivacaftor vs Placebo) in the first part of the study (+1.7 percentage points, $p = 0.15$), but a very small reduction in sweat chloride levels was observed (−2.9 mmol/L, $p = 0.04$). These changes were not maintained in the open-label phase. The safety profile of ivacaftor was similar to that of placebo with no new concerns raised. This study was demonstrated that ivacaftor as a CFTR potentiator alone is not beneficial as monotherapy in CF patients homozygous for the F508del mutation. That's why, additional therapy is required to restore functional CFTR to patients who have class II mutations or quantitative defects in protein presence at the epithelial cell surface. CFTR correctors are a mediator designed to assist the protein folding in intra-cellular and trafficking to the cell surface. In vitro, studies have suggested that the CFTR correctors can restore maturation, but the addition of a potentiator of CFTR has significantly increased chloride transport, indicating that 'corrected' mutant CFTR has a gating defect that needs to be additionally targeted to restore chloride conductance (Van Goor et al., 2011). This finding has led to the current strategy of targeting class II mutations with a combined CFTR 'corrector' and 'potentiator' approach.

Lumacaftor (VX-809) is the most frequent CFTR corrector studied. Using an approach similar to the discovery of ivacaftor, 164,000 small molecules were screened in cell-based assays and VX-809, later known as lumacaftor, was identified as a lead compound (Van Goor et al., 2011). His chemical named is 3-[6-(amino)-3-methylpyridin-2-yl] benzoic acid, or C24H18F2N2O5 (Figure 2). Lumacaftor improves the conformational stability of F508del-CFTR, which ultimately increases the total amount of CFTR at the cell surface. The half-life of lumacaftor is approximately 26 hours in patients with CF, and it is almost entirely bound to plasma proteins.

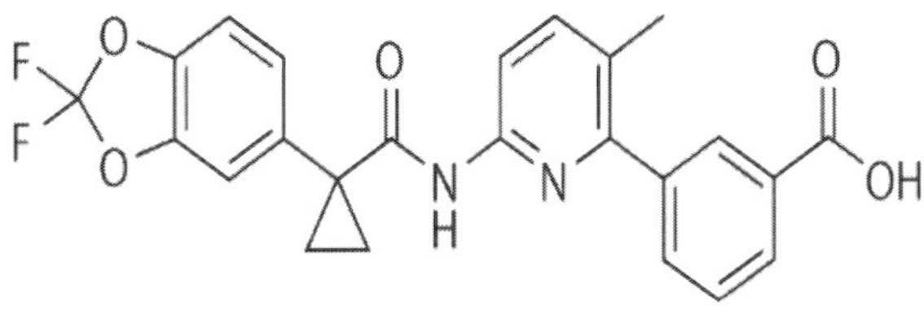

Figure 2. Lumacaftor.

In vitro studies have shown that lumacaftor improves CFTR processing and chloride secretion in bronchial epithelial cells derived from people with cystic fibrosis homozygous for F508del (Van Goor et al., 2011).

In phase II of clinical trials a randomized, double-blind, placebo-controlled trial that enrolled adult CF patients, homozygous for the F508del, into one of four once daily doses of lumacaftor (25, 50, 100, 200 mg) compared with placebo for 28 days (Clancy et al., 2012). Treatment with lumacaftor had a similar safety and adverse event profile to treatment with placebo and no major safety concerns were raised. Modest but statistically significant dose-dependent improvements in sweat chloride levels were demonstrated with lumacaftor treatment. Clinical efficacy measures (lung function, pulmonary exacerbations, and CFQ-R outcomes) and other CFTR biomarkers (nasal potential difference and mature C Band CFTR protein detection in rectal biopsies) did not differ significantly from placebo controls in those administered lumacaftor (Clancy et al., 2012). This study did not lead to clinical benefits for the patients under study, further emphasising the need for the addition of a CFTR potentiator to restore CFTR function. This approach was tested in a further phase II trial and the result is a relative improvement in lung function amongst F508del homozygotes in two dosing cohorts, with a modest decrease in sweat chloride measurements.

In phase II trial of combinated therapy (Ivacaftor + Lucaftor) was conducted in adult CF patients with two copies of the F508del CFTR mutation and placebo. The purpose of this study was to investigating the effects of varying doses of lumacaftor in combination with ivacaftor versus placebo (Boyle et al., 2014). The trial contain three successive cohorts of participants, with the results of earlier cohorts informing optimal dosing of lumacaftor for subsequent ones. The first cohort consisted of 64 F508del homozygous patients, and the second and third cohorts included 96 homozygotes and 28 compound heterozygotes. The primary outcomes were change in sweat chloride levels and safety, with secondary outcomes including percentage predicted FEV1. A modest yet statistically significant reduction in sweat chloride levels was demonstrated in treatment groups compared with placebo groups, as well as an increase of 5.6 percentage points in predicted FEV1 in the highest lumacaftor dose group. There was no significant change in FEV1 in the compound heterozygous subgroup. The frequency and nature of adverse events were similar between treatment and placebo groups, with no new concerns raised during the study. A large multi-national phase III trial of lumacaftor and ivacaftor combination therapy involving two dosing cohorts. Each cohort was randomized, double-blinded and placebo-controlled, and recruited patients aged ≥12 years who were homozygous for F508del. Participants were randomized to receive placebo or one of two different lumacaftor doses (400 mg twice daily or 600 mg once daily) and ivacaftor (250 mg twice daily). Significant improvements in FEV1 (2.6–4.0% absolute change) was conducted in the treatment groups. In addition, patients receiving combination therapy had a significantly lower rate of pulmonary exacerbations and a small but statistically significant increase in body mass index when pooled data were examined. In terms of CFQ-R, a significant improvement in pooled analyses was only observed for the for the 600 mg once-daily lumacaftor treatment group (Wainwright et al., 2015). Each of the dosing regimens of lumacaftor seemed to have similar efficacy, with the exception of pulmonary exacerbation outcomes, which were more favorable in the 400 mg twice-daily lumacaftor group. Lumacaftor combined with ivacaftor for F508del homozygous was recently approved by the US Food and Drug administration and by the European Medicines Agency, and is currently under review in Canada and Australia.

VX-661 is another orally administered CFTR corrector small-molecule drug. Although similar mechanistically to lumacaftor, it offers the potential benefits of a longer halflife and lower potential for drug interactions (Donaldson et al., 2013). In vivo, the combination of VX-661/Ivacaftor has been reported to improve trafficking and processing CFTR protein in patiens heterozygous for F508del/G551D mutations. In North American Cystic Fibrosis Conference, a blinded, randomized and placebo-controlled, and involved different dosing regimensstudy was reported the safety of VX-661and a change in sweat chloride levels after 28 days of treatment (Pilewski et al., 2014). Futur study are necessary for the determination of effectiveness of the VX-661.

Targeted Therapies for Patients with Class I Mutation

Ataluren, formerly known as PTC124, (3-(5-(2-fluorophenyl)-1,2,4-oxadiazol-3-yl)-benzoic acid) is an orally bioavailable agent that has been trialed for use in class I CFTR mutations (Figure 3). Ataluren is structurally similar to the aminoglycoside antibiotic gentamicin in terms of its functional properties but he does not have the antibiotic characteristics or toxicity of an aminoglycoside (Hamed, 2006; Ratjen, 2009). Using a stable cell line, ataluren was shown to be a 4- to 15-fold more potent read-through agent relative to controls (Welch et al., 2007). Ataluren was recently approved by the European Medicine agency with an 'orphan designation' as a treatment for Duchenne Muscular Dystrophy and is supplied by the name Translarna (Rowe et al., 2005).

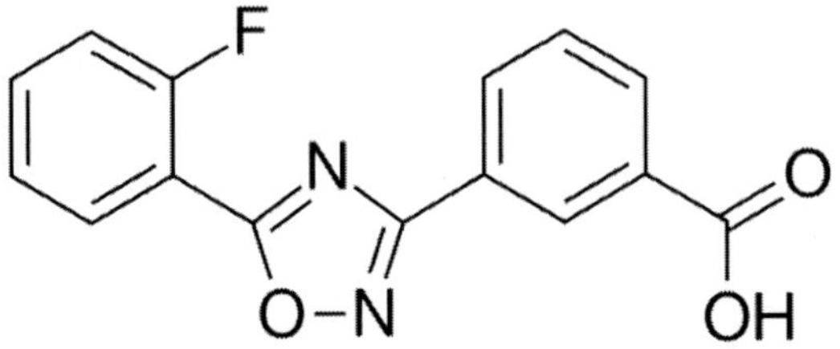

Figure 3. Ataluren.

A phase II prospective clinical trial of ataluren was performed in adult patients with cystic fibrosis and a class I CFTR mutation; the trial included 23 participants in the first cycle and 21 in the second (Kerem et al., 2014). Each cycle varied in the dose of ataluren used but involved 14 days of treatment, with assessment of CFTR-mediated chloride transport by measurements of the transepithelial nasal potential difference. There was no placebo group. Oral treatment with ataluren was associated with an improvement in electrophysiological profile in the majority of patients. In 13 patients in cycle 1 and 9 patients in cycle 2, total chloride transport entered the normal range. Ataluren was generally well tolerated by the study participants. A further 19 patients entered a follow-on study, in which they received varying doses of ataluren for another 12 weeks. The results of this study showed ongoing improvement in CFTR function as assessed by evaluation of the nasal potential difference and raised no new safety issues (Wilschanski et al., 2007). This study was replicated in young patients aged between 6 and 18 years with a class I mutation, the primary outcome was nasal potential difference. In around half of the participants an electrophysiological response was demonstrated with ataluren treatment and the agent was generally well tolerated (Sermet-Gaudelus et al., 2010). In phase III trial, the 238 patients were recruited and randomized to receive placebo or ataluren for 48 weeks. The primary outcome was change in percentage predicted FEV1, with the number of pulmonary exacerbations as a secondary outcome. There was no statistically significant difference between ataluren treatment and placebo for the primary outcome. The secondary outcome was also not statistically significantly different between the two groups. A post hoc analysis was performed in patients not taking inhaled tobramycin regularly. The analysis showed that this group had a significant increase in FEV1 of around 5% with ataluren treatment compared with placebo (−0.7% versus −6.4%, P=0.0082), along with a reduction in the number of pulmonary exacerbations (Kerem et al., 2014). The authors concluded that the drug may be of benefit to those not receiving inhaled tobramycin treatment, but it should be noted that, to date, no phase III trial of ataluren in cystic fibrosis has met its endpoints (Kerem et al., 2014). It has been hypothesized that tobramycin interferes with the mechanism of action of (Kerem et al., 2 014), and a further phase III study is underway to investigate the efficacy of ataluren in patients not receiving this antibiotic (ClinicalTrials.gov identifier NCT02139306) (Brodlie et al., 2015).

Other CFTR modulator are currently under investigation (Figure 4). However, major challenges lie ahead to demonstrate longer-term benefits of these drugs, to develop compounds that target the most common classes of CFTR mutations.

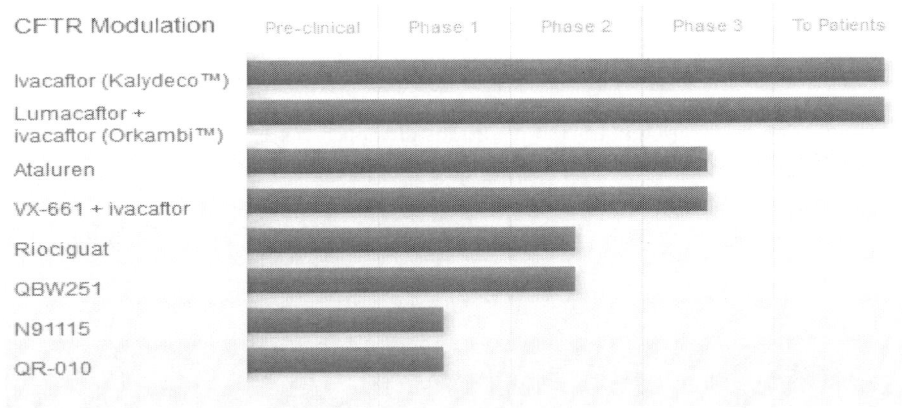

Figure 4. CFTR modilator (Cystic Fibrosis Fondation, 2016).

GENE THERAPY

Since the discovery of the CFTR gene in 1989, the restoration of wild-type CFTR DNA into human epithelial cells and to restore functional CFTR protein to all patients with CF has been a focus of CF research. The cloning of CFTR gene in 1989 and thefirst studies of opened the door for the development of cystic fibrosis (CF) gene therapy. Gene therapy has been described as "the introduction or alteration of genetic material within a cell or organism with the intentions of curing or treating a disease" (American Society of Cell and Gene Therapy, 2011). The earliest clinical trials in CF patients were conducted in 1993 and used viral and non-viral gene transfer agents in both the nasal and bronchial airway epithelium (Burney et Davies, 2012). In 2001, the UK Cystic Fibrosis Gene Therapy Consortium http://www.cfgenetherapy.org.uk/) was created, with the aim of coordinating gene therapy in the UK. Recently, a randomized, double-blind, placebo-controlled, phase 2b trial was conducted to assess the clinical efficacy of a non-viral CFTR gene-liposome complex (pGM169/GL67A) as a delivery system for a functional CFTR gene in the airways of patients with CF (Alton et al., 2015). This study included 136 CF patients aged 12 and above were randomly assigned to either 5 ml of nebulised pGM169/GL67A (gene therapy) or saline (placebo) at monthly intervals over one year. Patients receiving therapy have a modest improvement in lung function compared with those receiving a placebo (Alton et al., 2015). After a year of treatment, in the 62 patients who received the gene therapy, FEV1 was 3.7% greater compared to placebo. This study is the first ever to show that repeated doses of a gene therapy can have a meaningful effect on the disease and change the lung function of patients. A truncated version of the CFTR gene that retained function can be transfected using adenovirus-associated viral vectors and restored CFTR function in a CF mouse model as well as ex vivo in patient tissue was producted (Carlon et al., 2015). Compared to the target therapy the advantage of the gene therapy approach is its potential use in all mutation classes.

Conclusion

Over the past few decades, remarkable improvements have been made in clinical outcomes for CF patients including better nutritional status, new target and gene therapy. Many drug have also been developed to improve the quality of life of patients. The *researchers* challenge is to find and improve therapies in order to enhance morbidity and mortality in CF.

References

Accurso, F.J., Rowe, S.M., Clancy, J.P., Boyle, M.P., Dunitz, J.M., Durie, P.R., Sagel, S.D., Hornick, D.B., Konstan, M.W., Donaldson, S.H., Moss, R.B., Pilewski, J.M., Rubenstein, R.C., Uluer, A.Z., Aitken, M.L., Freedman, S.D., Rose, L.M., Mayer-Hamblett, N., Dong, Q., Zha, J., Stone, A.J., Olson, E.R., Ordoñez, C.L., Campbell, P.W., Ashlock, M.A.,

Ramsey, B.W. 2010. Effect of VX-770 in persons with cystic fibrosis and the G551D-CFTR mutation. *N Engl J Med,* 18,363(21):1991-2003.

Agent, P., Parrott, H. (2015). Inhaled therapy in cystic fibrosis: agents, devices and regimens. *Breathe* (Sheff), 11(2):110-8.

Alton, E.W., Armstrong, D.K., Ashby, D., Bayfield, K.J., Bilton, D., Bloomfield, E.V., Boyd, A.C., Brand, J., Buchan, R., Calcedo, R., Carvelli, P., Chan, M., Cheng, S.H., Collie, D.D., Cunningham, S., Davidson, H.E., Davies, G., Davies, J.C., Davies, L.A., Dewar, M.H., Doherty, A., Donovan, J., Dwyer, N.S., Elgmati, H.I., Featherstone, R.F., Gavino, J., Gea-Sorli, S., Geddes, D.M., Gibson, J.S., Gill, D.R., Greening, A.P., Griesenbach, U, Hansell, D.M., Harman, K., Higgins, T.E., Hodges, S.L., Hyde, S.C., Hyndman, L., Innes, J.A., Jacob, J., Jones, N., Keogh, B.F., Limberis, M.P., Lloyd-Evans, P., Maclean, A.W., Manvell, M.C., McCormick, D., McGovern, M., McLachlan, G., Meng, C., Montero, M.A., Milligan, H., Moyce, L.J., Murray, G.D., Nicholson, A.G., Osadolor, T., Parra-Leiton, J., Porteous, D.J., Pringle, I.A., Punch, E.K., Pytel, K.M., Quittner, A.L., Rivellini, G., Saunders, C.J., Scheule, R.K., Sheard, S., Simmonds, N.J., Smith, K., Smith, S.N., Soussi, N., Soussi, S., Spearing, E.J., Stevenson, B.J., Sumner-Jones, S.G., Turkkila, M., Ureta, R.P., Waller, M.D., Wasowicz, M.Y., Wilson, J.M., Wolstenholme-Hogg, P., UK Cystic Fibrosis Gene Therapy Consortium. (2015). Repeated nebulisation of non-viral CFTR gene therapy in patients with cystic fibrosis: a randomised, double-blind, placebo-controlled, phase 2b trial. *Lancet Respir Med,* 3(9):684-91.

Amaral, M.D. and Kunzelmann, K. Molecular targeting of CFTR as a therapeutic approach to cystic fibrosis. (2007). TRENDS in *Pharmacological Sciences,* 28(7): 334-341.

American Society of Cell and Gene Therapy. Gene Therapy Defined. Secondary Gene.

Barry, P.J., Plant, B.J., Nair, A., Bicknell, S., Simmonds, N.J., Bell, N.J., Shafi, N.T., Daniels, T., Shelmerdine, S., Felton, I., Gunaratnam, C., Jones, A.M., Horsley, A.R. (2014). Effects of ivacaftor in patients with cystic fibrosis who carry the G551D mutation and have severe lung disease. *Chest,* 146:152–8.

Bosch, B. and Boeck, K.D. (2016). Searching for a cure for cystic fibrosis. A 25-year quest in a nutshell. *Eur J Pediatr,* 175(1):1-8.

Boyle, M.P., Bell, S.C., Konstan, M.W., McColley, S.A., Rowe, S.M., Rietschel, E., Huang, X., Waltz, D., Patel, N.R., Rodman, D.,VX09-809-102 study group. (2014). A CFTR corrector (lumacaftor) and a CFTR potentiator (ivacaftor) for treatment of patients with cystic fibrosis who have a phe508del CFTR mutation: a phase 2 randomised controlled trial. *Lancet Respir Med,* 2(7):527–38.

Boyle, M.P., Boeck, K.D. (2013). A new era in the treatment of cystic fi brosis: correction of the underlying CFTR defect. *Lancet Resp Med,* 1: 158–63.

Brodlie, M., Haq, I.J., Roberts, K., Elborn, J.S. (2015). Targeted therapies to improve CFTR function in cystic fibrosis. *Genome Med,* 24;7(1):101.

Burney, T.J., and Davies J.C. (2012). Gene therapy for the treatment of cystic fibrosis. *Appl Clin Genet,* 5: 29–36.

Bush, A., Alton, E.W.F.W., Davies, J.C., Griesenbach, U., Jaffe, A.(2006). Cystic Fibrosis in the 21st Century. *Prog Respir Res. Basel Karger,* 34: 293-300.

Cai, Z.W., Liu, J., Li, H.Y., Sheppard, D.N. (2011). Targeting F508del-CFTR to develop rational new therapies for cystic fibrosis. *Acta Pharmacol Sin,* 32:693–701.

Carlon, M.S., Vidovic, D., Dekkers, J.F., Faria da Cunha, M., Hollenhorst, M.I., Bijvelds, M., Van den Haute, C., Baekelandt, V., de Jonge, H., De Boeck, K., Gijsbers, R., Sermet-Gaudelus, I., Edelman, A., Beekman, J., Debyser, Z. (2015). WS01.1 rAAV2/5 encoding a truncated CFTR rescues the CF phenotype in intestinal organoids and a CFmousemodel. *J Cyst Fibros,* 14(1):S1.

Clancy, J.P., Jain, M. (2012). Personalized medicine in cystic fibrosis: dawning of a new era. *Am J Respir Crit Care Med,* 186: 593–597.

Clancy, J.P., Rowe, S.M., Accurso, F.J., Aitken, M.L., Amin, R.S., Ashlock, M.A., Ballmann, M., Boyle, M.P., Bronsveld, I., Campbell, P.W., De Boeck, K., Donaldson, S.H., Dorkin, H.L., Dunitz, J.M., Durie, P.R., Jain, M., Leonard, A., McCoy, K.S., Moss, R.B., Pilewski, J.M., Rosenbluth, D.B., Rubenstein, R.C., Schechter, M.S., Botfield, M., Ordoñez, C.L., Spencer-Green, G.T., Vernillet, L., Wisseh, S., Yen, K., Konstan, M.W. (2012). Results of a phase IIa study of VX-809, an investigational CFTR corrector compound, in subjects with cystic fibrosis homozygous for the F508del-CFTR mutation. *Thorax,* 67(1):12-8.

Collins, F.S. (1992). Cystic fibrosis: molecular biology and therapeutic implications. *Science,* 256: 774–779.

Collins, F.S., Varmus, H. (2015). A new initiative on precision medicine. *N Engl J Med,* 372:793–5.

Cuppens, H., Cassiman,J.J. (2004). CFTR mutations and polymorphisms in male infertility. *Int J Androl,* 27:251–256.

Dames, P., Gleich, B., Flemmer, A., Hajek, K., Seidl, N., Wiekhorst, F., Eberbeck, D., Bittmann, I., Bergemann, C., Weyh, T., Trahms, L., Rosenecker, J., Rudolph, C. (2007). Targeted delivery of magnetic aerosol droplets to the lung. *Nat Nanotechnol*, 2(8):495–499 122.

Davies, J.C., Wainwright, C.E., Canny, G.J., Chilvers, M.A., Howenstine, M.S., Munck, A., Mainz, J.G., Rodriguez, S., Li, H., Yen, K., Ordoñez, C.L., Ahrens, R., VX08-770-103 (ENVISION) Study Group. (2013). Efficacy and safety of ivacaftor in patients aged 6 to 11 years with cystic fibrosis with a G551D mutation. *Am J Respir Crit Care Med,* 187(11):1219–25.

Davis, P.B., Drumm, M., Konstan, M.W. (1996). Cystic fibrosis. *Am J Respir Crit Care Med,* 154(5):1229–56.

De Boeck, K., Munck, A., Walker, S., Faro, A., Hiatt, P., Gilmartin, G., Higgins, M. (2014). Efficacy and safety of ivacaftor in patients with cystic fibrosis and a non-G551D gating mutation. *J Cyst Fibros,* 13(6):674-80.

Denning, G., Ostedgaard, L., Welsh, M. (1992) Abnormal localization of cystic fibrosis transmembrane conductance regulator in primary cultures of cystic fibrosis airway epithelia. *J Cell Biol,* 118(3): 551–559.

Donaldson, S., Pilewski, J., Griese, M., Dong, Q., Lee, P.S. WS7. (2013). 3VX-661, an investigational CFTR corrector, in combination with ivacaftor, a CFTR potentiator, in patients with CF and homozygous for the F508Del-CFTR mutation: interim analysis. *J Cyst Fibros,* 12(S1):S14.

Drug Development Pipeline, 2016. https://tools.cff.org/research/Drug DevelopmentPipeline/.

Durmowicz, A.G., Witzmann, K.A., Rosebraugh, C.J., Chowdhury, B.A. (2013). Change in sweat chloride as a clinical end point in cystic fibrosis clinical trials: the ivacaftor experience. *Chest,* 143(1):14-8.

Eckford, P.D., Li, C., Ramjeesingh, M., Bear, C.E. (2012). Cystic fibrosis transmembrane conductance regulator (CFTR) potentiator VX-770 (ivacaftor) opens the defective channel gate of mutant CFTR in a phosphorylation-dependent but ATP-independent manner. *J Biol Chem,* 287:36639–36649.

Fanen, P., Wohlhuter-Haddad, A., Hinzpeter, A. (2014). Genetics of cystic fibrosis: CFTR mutation classifications toward genotype-based CF therapies. *Int J Biochem Cell Biol,* 52:94-102.

Fieker,A., Philpott, J., Armand, M. (2011). Enzyme replacement therapy for pancreatic insuciency: present and future. Clinical and Experimental Gastroenterology, *Dove Medical Press,* 4 (4), 55-73.

Fiel, S.B. (2014). Aerosolized antibiotics in cystic fibrosis: an update *Expert Rev. Respir. Med,* 8(3):305–314.

Flume, P.A. (2009). Pulmonary complications of cystic fibrosis. *Respir Care,* 54(5): 618-27.

Flume, P.A., Liou, T.G., Borowitz, D.S., Li, H., Yen, K., Ordonez, C.L., Geller, D.E. (2012). Ivacaftor in subjects with cystic fibrosis who are homozygous for the F508del-CFTR mutation. *Chest,* 142:718–24.

Geus, W.P., Gan, K.H., Lamers, C.B.H.W., Heijerman, H.G.M. (1999). Simultaneously measured duodenal and gastric pH in patients with cystic fibrosis: effect of omeprazole. *Neth J Med* [Suppl], 54:63.

Gilbert, J., Kelleher, J., Littlewood, J.M., Evans, D.F. (1988). Ileal pH in cystic fibrosis. *Scand J Gastroenterol* [Suppl 143], 23:132–134.

Haardt, M., Benharouga, M., Lechardeur, D., Kartner, N., Lukacs, G.L. (1999). C-terminal truncations destabilize the cystic fibrosis transmembrane conductance regulator without impairing its biogenesis. A novel class of mutation. *J Biol Chem,* 274(31):21873-7.

Haardt, M., Benharouga, M., Lechardeur, D., Kartner, N., Lukacs, G.L. (1999). C-terminal Truncations Destabilize the Cystic Fibrosis Transmembrane Conductance Regulator without Impairing Its Biogenesis. *Journal of Biological Chemistry,* 274 (31): 21873–21877.

Hall, I.P. (2013). Stratified medicine: drugs meet genetics. *Eur Respir Rev.* 22:53–7.

Hamed, S.A. (2006). Drug evaluation: PTC-124: a potential treatment of cystic fibrosis and Duchenne muscular dystrophy. *IDrugs,* 9:783–789.

Heijerman H, Westerman, E., Conway, S., Touw, D., Döring, G.,consensus working group. (2009). Inhaled medication and inhalation devices for lung disease in patients with cystic fibrosis: a European consensus. *J Cyst Fibros,* 8: 295–315.

Hodson, M.E., Penketh, A.R.L., Batten, J.C. (1981). Aerosol carbenicillin and gentamicin treatment of Pseudomonas aeruginosa in patients with cystic fibrosis. *Lancet,* 2: 1137–113.

Kalivianakis, M., Minich, D.M., Bijleveld, C.M.A., van Aalderen, W.M., Stellaard, F., Laseur, M. (1999). Fat malabsorption in cystic fibrosis patients receiving enzyme replacement therapy is due to impaired intestinal uptake of long chain fatty acids. *Am J Clin Nutr,* 69:127–134.

Kerem, E., Konstan, M.W., De Boeck, K., Accurso, F.J., Sermet-Gaudelus, I., Wilschanski, M., Elborn, J.S., Melotti, P., Bronsveld, I., Fajac, I., Malfroot, A., Rosenbluth, D.B., Walker, P.A., McColley, S.A., Knoop,C., Quattrucci, S., Rietschel, E., Zeitlin, P.L., Barth, J., Elfring, G.L., Welch,

E.M., Branstrom, A., Spiegel, R.J., Peltz, S.W., Ajayi, T., Rowe, S.M., Cystic Fibrosis Ataluren Study Group. (2014). Ataluren for the treatment of non sense mutation cystic fibrosis: A randomised, double-blind, placebo-controlled phase 3 trial. *Lancet Respir Med,* 2:539-47.

Kuk, K., Taylor-Cousar, J.L. (2015). Lumacaftor and ivacaftor in the management of patients with cystic fibrosis: current evidence and future prospects. *Ther Adv Respir Dis*, 9(6):313-26.

Laiho, K.M., Gavin, J., Murphy, J.L., Connett, G.J., Stephen, S.A., Wootton, S. (2004). Maldigestion and malabsorption of 13 C labelled tripalmitin in gastrostomy-fed patients with cystic fibrosis. *Clin Nutr,* 23:347–353.

Ledford, H. (2012). Drug bests cystic-fibrosis mutation. *Nature,* 482:145.

Littlewood, J.M., Wolfe, S.P., Conway, S.P. (2006). Diagnosis and treatment of intestinal malabsorption in cystic fibrosis. *Pediatr Pulmonol*, 41: 35-49.

Manca, M.L., Cassano, R., Valenti, D., Trombino, S., Ferrarelli, T., Picci, N., Fadda, A.M., Manconi, M. (2013). Isoniazid-gelatin conjugate microparticles containing rifampicin for the treatment of tuberculosis. *J Pharm Pharmacol,* 65(9):1302–1311.

Maquat, L.E. (1995). When cells stop making sense: effects of nonsense codons on RNAmetabolism in vertebrate cells. *RNA,* 1:453–65.

McKone, E.F., Borowitz, D., Drevinek, P., Griese, M., Konstan, M.W., Wainwright, C., Ratjen, F., Sermet-Gaudelus, I., Plant, B., Munck, A., Jiang, Y., Gilmartin, G., Davies, J.C., VX08-770-105 (PERSIST) Study Group. (2014). Long-term safety and efficacy of ivacaftor in patients with cystic fibrosis who have the Gly551Asp- CFTR mutation: a phase 3, open-label extension study (PERSIST). *Lancet Respir Med.,* 2(11):902–10.

Mogayzel, P.J. Jr, Naureckas, E.T., Robinson, K.A., Mueller, G., Hadjiliadis, D., Hoag, J.B., Lubsch, L., Hazle, L., Sabadosa, K., Marshall, B.,Pulmonary Clinical Practice Guidelines Committee. (2013). Cystic fibrosis pulmonary guidelines. Chronic medications for maintenance of lung health. *Am J Respir Crit Care Med,* 187(7):680–9.

No authors listed. (1990). Worldwide survey of the delta F508 mutation – report from the cystic fibrosis genetic analysis consortium. *Am J Hum Genet,* 47: 354–359.

O'Reilly, R., Elphick, H.E. (2013). Development, clinical utility, and place of ivacaftor in the treatment of cystic fibrosis. *Drug Design, Development and Therapy,* 7 929–937.

Park, J., Khloya, P., Seo, Y., Kumar, S., Lee, H.K., Jeon, D.K., Jo, S., Sharma, P.K., Namkung, W.(2016). Potentiation of ΔF508- and G551D-CFTR-

Mediated Cl- Current by Novel Hydroxypyrazolines. *PLoS One,* 10;11(2):e0149131.

Pilewski, J.M., Donaldson, S.H., Cooke, J., Lekstrom-Himes, J.(2014). Phase 2 studies reveal additive effects of VX-661, an investigational CFTR corrector and ivacaftor, a CFTR potentiator, in patients with CF who carry the d508-CFTR mutation. *Ped Pulmonol,* 49:157.

Plank, C. (2008). Nanomagnetosols: magnetism opens up new perspectives for targeted aerosol delivery to the lung. Trends Biotechnol, 26(2):59–63.

Product information. Kalydeco (ivacaftor). Cambridge, MA: Vertex Pharmaceuticals Inc., January 2012.

Ramsey, B.W., Davies, J., McElvaney, G., Tullis, E., Bell, S.C., Dřevínek, P., Griese, M., McKone, E.F., Wainwright,C.E,. Konstan, M.W., Moss, R., Ratjen, F., Sermet-Gaudelus, I., Rowe, S.M., Dong, Q., Rodriguez, S., Yen, K., Ordoñez, C., Elborn, J.S., for the VX08-770-102 Study Group. (2011). A CFTR Potentiator in Patients with Cystic Fibrosis and the G551D Mutation. *N Engl J Med,* 365 (18):1663-1672.

Ramsey, B.W., Davies, J., McElvaney, N.G., Tullis, E., Bell, S.C., Dřevínek, P., Griese, M., McKone, E.F., Wainwright, C.E., Konstan, M.W., Moss, R., Ratjen, F., Sermet-Gaudelus, I., Rowe, S.M., Dong, Q., Rodriguez, S., Yen, K., Ordoñez, C., Elborn, J.S., VX08-770-102 Study Group. (2011). A CFTR potentiator in patients with cystic fibrosis and the G551D mutation. *N Engl J Med,* 365:1663–1672.

Ratjen, F.A. (2009). Cystic fibrosis: Pathogenesis and future treatment strategies. *Respir Care,* 54:595–602.

Rogan, M.P., Stoltz, D.A., Hornick, D.B. (2011). Cystic fibrosis transmembrane conductance regulator intracellular processing, trafficking, and opportunities for mutation-specific treatment. *Chest,* 139:1480–1490.

Rowe, S.M., Miller, S., Sorscher, E.J.(2005). Cystic Fibrosis. *N Engl J Med,* 352:1992-2001.

Roy, C.C., Weber, A.M., Morin, C.L., Combes, J.C., Nusslé, D., Mégevand, A., Lasalle, R. (1977). Abnormal biliary composition in cystic fibrosis. Effect of pancreatic enzymes. *N Engl J Med,* 297: 1301–1305.

Sermet-Gaudelus, I., Boeck, K.D., Casimir, G.J., Vermeulen, F., Leal, T., Mogenet, A., Roussel, D., Fritsch, J., Hanssens, L., Hirawat, S., Miller, N.L., Constantine, S., Reha, A., Ajayi, T., Elfring, G.L., Miller, L.L.(2010). Ataluren (PTC124) induces cystic fibrosis transmembrane conductance regulator protein expression and activity in children with nonsense mutation cystic fibrosis. *Am J Resp Crit Care Med*, 182:1262–72.

Sinaasappel, M.(1992). Relationship between intestinal function and chloride secretion in patients with cystic fibrosis. *Neth J Med*, 41:110–114.

Smyth, A.R., Bell, S.C., Bojcin, S., Bryon, M., Duff, A., Flume, P., Kashirskaya, N., Munck, A., Ratjen, F., Schwarzenberg, S.J., Sermet-Gaudelus, I., Southern, K.W., Taccetti, G., Ullrich, G., Wolfe, S., European Cystic Fibrosis Society. (2014). European cystic fibrosis society standards of care: best practice guidelines. *J Cyst Fibros,* 13(S1):S23–42.

Study of Ataluren in Nonsense Mutation Cystic Fibrosis (ACT CF). https://clinicaltrials.gov/ct2/show/NCT02139306.

Therapy Defined 2011. http://www.asgct.org/about_gene_therapy/defined.php.

Thomas, P., Ko, Y., Pedersen, P. (1992) Altered protein folding may be the molecular basis of most cases of cystic fibrosis. *FEBS Lett,* 312: 7–9.

Trang, T., Chan, J., Graham, D.Y. (2014). Pancreatic enzyme replacement therapy for pancreatic exocrine insufficiency in the 21St century. *World J Gastroenterol,* 20(33): 11467-11485.

Van Goor, F., Hadida, S., Grootenhuis, P.D., Burton, B., Cao, D., Neuberger, T., Turnbull, A., Singh, A., Joubran, J., Hazlewood, A., Zhou, J., McCartney, J., Arumugam, V., Decker, C., Yang, J., Young, C., Olson, ER., Wine, J.J., Frizzell, R.A., Ashlock, M., Negulescu, P. (2009). Rescue of CF airway epithelial cell function in vitro by a CFTR potentiator, VX-770. *Proc Natl Acad Sci U S A,* 106(44):18825-30.

Van Goor, F., Hadida, S., Grootenhuis, P.D., Burton, B., Cao, D., Neuberger, T., Turnbull, A., Singh, A., Joubran, J., Hazlewood, A., Zhou, J., McCartney, J., Arumugam, V., Decker, C., Yang, J., Young, C., Olson, E.R., Wine, J.J., Frizzell, R.A., Ashlock, M., Negulescu, P. (2009). Rescue of CF airway epithelial cell function in vitro by a CFTR potentiator, VX-770. *Proc Natl Acad Sci U S A*, 106: 18825–18830.

Van Goor, F., Hadida, S., Grootenhuis, P.D., Burton, B., Stack, J.H., Straley, K.S., Decker, C.J., Miller, M., McCartney, J., Olson, E.R., Wine, J.J., Frizzell, R.A., Ashlock, M., Negulescu, P.A. (2011). Correction of the F508del-CFTR protein processing defect in vitro by the investigational drug VX-809. *Proc Natl Acad Sci*, 108(46):18843–8.

Van Goor, F., Straley, K.S., Cao, D., González, J., Hadida, S., Hazlewood, A., Joubran, J., Knapp, T.,Makings, L.R., Miller, M., Neuberger, T., Olson, E., Panchenko, V., Rader, J., Singh, A., Stack, J.H., Tung, R., Grootenhuis, P.D., Negulescu, P. (2006). Rescue of DeltaF508-CFTR trafficking and gating in human cystic fibrosis airway primary cultures by small molecules. *Am J Physiol Lung Cell Mol Physiol,* 290(6): L1117–30.

Vertex Pharmaceuticals. Vertex announces results of phase 3 study of ivacaftor in people with CF who have the R117H mutation. Dec 19, 2013. Available at: http://investors.vrtx.com/releasedetail.cfm?ReleaseID=814799. Accessed March 2, 2014.

Wainwright, C.E., Elborn, J.S., Ramsey, B.W. (2015). Lumacaftor–ivacaftor in patients with cystic fibrosis homozygous for Phe508del CFTR. *N Engl J Med,* 373(18):1783-4.

Walters, M.P. and Littlewood, J.M.(1998). Fecal bile acid and dietary residue excretion in cystic fibrosis: age group variations. *J Pediatr Gastroenterol Nutr,* 27:296–300.

Welch, E.M., Barton, E.R., Zhuo, J., Tomizawa, Y., Friesen, W.J., Trifillis, P., Paushkin, S., Patel, M., Trotta, C.R., Hwang, S., Wilde, R.G., Karp, G., Takasugi, J., Chen, G., Jones, S., Ren, H., Moon, Y.C., Corson, D., Turpoff, A.A., Campbell, J.A., Conn, M.M., Khan, A., Almstead, N.G., Hedrick, J., Mollin, A., Risher, N., Weetall, M., Yeh, S., Branstrom, A.A., Colacino, J.M., Babiak, J., Ju, W.D., Hirawat, S., Northcutt, V.J., Miller, L.L., Spatrick, P., He, F., Kawana, M., Feng, H., Jacobson, A., Peltz, S.W., Sweeney, H.L.(2007). PTC124 targets genetic disorders caused by nonsense mutations. *Nature,* 447: 87–91.

Welsh, M.J., Ramsey, B.W., Accurso, F., Cutting, G.R. (2013) Cystic fibrosis. Edited by Valle D, Beauder A, Vogelstein B, Kinzler KW, Antonarakis SE, Bellabio A, Gibson K, Mitchell G. OMMBID: the Online Metabolic and Molecular Basis of Inherited Diseases. New York, NY McGraw-Hill; 2013.

Wilschanski, M., Miller, L.L., Shoseyov, D., Blau, H., Rivlin, J., Aviram, M., Cohen, M., Armoni, S., Yaakov, Y., Pugatsch, T., Cohen-Cymberknoh, M., Miller, N.L., Reha, A., Northcutt, V.J., Hirawat, S., Donnelly, K., Elfring, G.L., Ajayi, T., Kerem, E. (2011). Chronic ataluren (PTC124) treatment of nonsense mutation cystic fibrosis. *Eur Respir J,* 38:59–69.

Yu, H., Burton, B., Huang, C.J., Worley, J., Cao, D., Johnson, J.P. Jr, Urrutia, A., Joubran, J., Seepersaud, S., Sussky, K., Hoffman, B.J., Van Goor, F. (2012). Ivacaftor potentiation of multiple CFTR channels with gating mutations. *J Cyst Fibros,* 11(3):237-45.

Zielenski, J., Tsui, L.P. (1995). Cystic fibrosis: genotype and phenotype variations. *Annual,* 29:777-807.

Biographical Sketch

Name: Sabrine Oueslati

Affiliation: Biochemistry Laboratory, Children's Hospital; Research laboratory "Haemoglobinopathies and Cystic fibrosis, LR00SP03", Tunis, Tunisia.

Education: PHD in Biology

Address: The Children's Hospital Bechir Hamza, Tunis,Tunisia Bab saadoun square

Research and Professional Experience: As a researcher, she's the author and the co-authors of several papers in peer-reviewed scientific journals. She has contributed to the organization and animation of many workshops and she has participated at several scientific meetings.

Professional Appointments: Researcher at the Research laboratory "Haemoglobinopathies and Cystic fibrosis, LR00SP03, Children's Hospital Bechir Hamza

Publications Last 3 Years:

OUESLATI Sabrine, HADJ Fredj Sondess, SIALA Hajer, BIBI Amina, ALOULOU Hajer, BOUGHAMOURA Lamia, BOUSSETTA Khadija, BARSAOUI Sihem, MESSAOUD Taieb. "Angiotensin-Converting Enzyme Insertion/Deletion Gene Polymorphism in cystic fibrosis patients", accepted in Journal of Genetis, 2015.

Oueslati Sabrine, Hadj Fredj Sondess, Dakhlaoui Bouthayna, Othmani Rim, Siala Hajer, Messaoud Taieb. "Association of TGFB1 -509C/T polymorphism gene with clinical variability in cystic fibrosis patients: A case-control study": in Pathologie Biologie Journal. 2015 Aug 13 doi: 10.1016/j.patbio.2015.07.003.

Oueslati Sabrine, Hadj Fredj S, Belhaj R, Siala H, Bibi A, Messaoud T. "Preliminary study of haplotypes linked to the rare cystic fibrosis E1104X mutation in a Tunisian population" in Acta Physiol Hung. Journal 2015 Mar;102(1):86-93.

Oueslati Sabrine, Hadj Fredj Sondess, Boudaya Monia, Sahli Chayma, Siala Hajer, Bibi Amina, Messaoud Taieb. "Etude des haplotypes associés à la mutation F508del dans une population Tunisienne", in Tunisian Journal RTBC 'Revue Tunisienne de Biologie Clinique', Vol 20, n° 1, 2013.

HADJ Hadj Fredj S, Boudaya M, Oueslati S, Sahnoun S, Sahli C, Siala H, Boussetta K, Bibi A, Messaoud T. " New frameshift CF mutation 3729delAinsTCT in a Tunisian cystic fibrosis patient." Journal of Genetics, 2013 Apr;92(1):81-3.

HADJ FREDJ Sondess, OUESLATI Sabrine, BOUDAYA Monia, SAHLI Chaima, SIALA Hajer, BIBI Amina, MESSAOUD Taieb. "Première description de la mutation mucoviscidosique R334W dans la population libyenne" RTBC (Tunisian national journal).

In: Cystic and Idiopathic Pulmonary Fibrosis
Editor: Lorenzo Robertson
ISBN: 978-1-63485-508-2

Chapter 5

DISTINCT PATTERNS OF PULMONARY INJURY AND FIBROSIS INDUCED BY INTRATRACHEAL AND SUBCUTANEOUS BLEOMYCIN IN THE MOUSE: RELEVANCE FOR DISTINCT FORMS OF HUMAN LUNG FIBROSIS

Anna P. Lam[2], Erica L. Herzog[4], Denisa Melichian[1], Joseph Sennello[2], Ye Gan[4], Kirtee Raparia[3], Robert Homer[4], Anjana Yeldandi[3] and John Varga[1,*]
[1]Divisions of Rheumatology,
[2]Pulmonary and Critical Care Medicine and
[3]Department of Pathology,
[4]Northwestern University Feinberg School of Medicine, Chicago, Illinois
Yale University School of Medicine,
New Haven, Connecticut, US

* Correspondence: John Varga, M.D., Department of Medicine, Division of Rheumatology, Feinberg School of Medicine, Northwestern University, 240 East Huron St., McGaw Pavilion, Chicago, IL 60611, Phone: (312) 503-8003, Fax: (312) 503-0994, email: j-varga@northwestern.edu.

ABSTRACT

Background: Murine models can be useful for understanding complex diseases such as pulmonary fibrosis. Bleomycin, administered via a wide variety of routes, is commonly used to induce lung fibrosis in rodents. We compared fibrotic responses in the lung elicited by bleomycin given by subcutaneous injection and intratracheal administration. Mice were treated with one dose of intratracheal bleomycin or with subcutaneous bleomycin daily for 14 days. Lungs and skin were analyzed for fibrosis by histopathology and immunostaining for alpha-smooth muscle actin, and transforming growth factor-beta protein level and apoptosis were evaluated. Results: While intratracheal and subcutaneous approaches yielded comparable severity of pulmonary fibrosis, distinct spatial and temporal evolution of pulmonary changes was noted. Intratracheal bleomycin induced early onset and rapid resolution of inflammation, while subcutaneous bleomycin caused more sustained lung inflammation with slow resolution of injury. Moreover, subcutaneous bleomcyin caused a predominantly peri-vascular pattern of lung fibrosis, whereas intratracheal instillation of bleomycin additionally caused injury around the airways. Early apoptotic responses were primarily centered around the airways in mice given intratracheal bleomycin but were seen around blood vessels with subcutaneous bleomycin. Conclusions: Subcutaneous administration of bleomycin causes a pattern of lung injury and fibrosis that is histologically distinct from that induced by the intratracheal route. These two distinct modes of bleomycin delivery might have utility for modeling interstitial lung disease associated with airway injury, such as idiopathic pulmonary fibrosis, versus systemic autoimmunity, such as systemic sclerosis.

Keywords: fibrosis, bleomycin, subcutaneous, intratracheal, mouse model, idiopathic pulmonary fibrosis, systemic sclerosis

LIST OF ABBREVIATIONS

Idiopathic Pulmonary Fibrosis (IPF);
Systemic Sclerosis-associated Interstitial Lung Disease (SSc-ILD);
Usual Interstitial Pneumonia (UIP);
Non-Specific Interstitial Pneumonia (NSIP).

INTRODUCTION

Pulmonary fibrosis can occur as an organ-restricted idiopathic entity or in association with systemic autoimmune diseases such as systemic sclerosis [1, 2]. In both forms, pulmonary fibrosis is characterized by excessive interstitial deposition of extracellular matrix and architectural distortion [3]. The pathogenesis of pulmonary fibrosis remains poorly understood [4, 5]. To study the mechanisms of pulmonary fibrogenesis, various murine models that recapitulate the fibrotic response have been utilized. Commonly used disease models include the administration of chemicals, such as bleomycin, fluorescein isothiocyanate (FITC), or silica; irradiation; transgenic gene expression or gene overexpression by viral vectors; and adoptive transfer of fibroblasts [reviewed in 6, 7]. Of these, fibrosis induced by bleomycin remains the most widely used [8]. An advantage of bleomycin for inducing pulmonary fibrosis is that it can be administered via intratracheal, intravenous, and intraperitoneal routes [9]. Recent studies have indicated that chronic subcutaneous administration of bleomycin can also induce pulmonary fibrosis in mice [10-13]. While the diverse routes of bleomycin administration all lead to the development of lung fibrosis, the differences in the associated pulmonary phenotypes and their ability to recapitulate diverse forms of human lung fibrosis have received scant attention to date.

To gain an understanding into the fibrotic phenotype induced by subcutaneous versus intratracheal bleomycin, we compared the effect of repetitive subcutaneous bleomycin administration to that of single intratracheal bleomycin instillation in parallel. The results show that fibrosis in the lungs induced by bleomycin displayed distinctive temporal and spatial patterns. In particular, subcutaneous bleomycin induced lung injury that was prominently centered around blood vessels, while intratracheal bleomycin caused injury that was focused additionally around airways. These differences in lung phenotypes may be exploited experimentally for investigating different aspects of human pulmonary fibrosis.

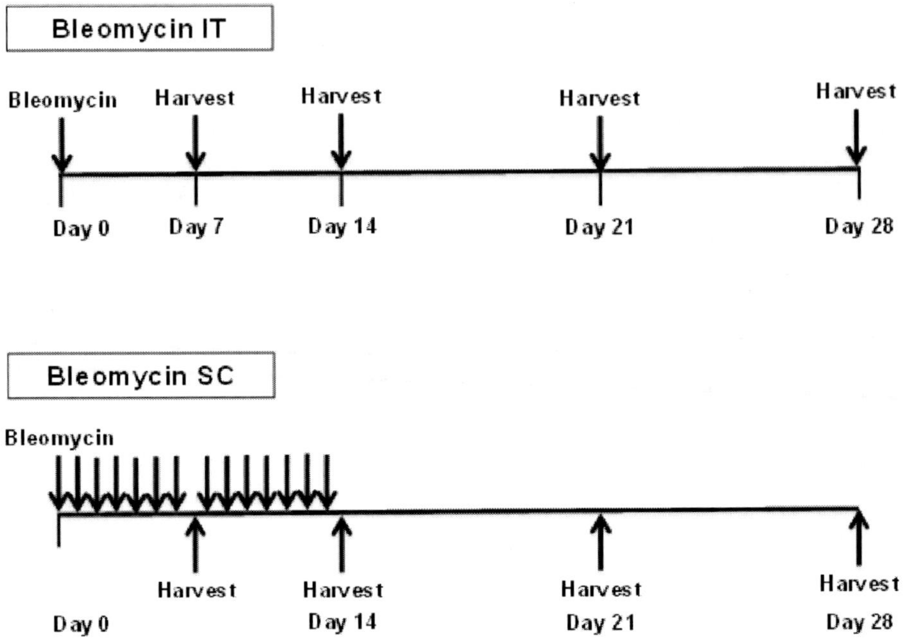

Figure 1. Strategy for administration of intratracheal and subcutaneous bleomycin.

RESULTS

Evolution of Injury and Fibrosis Induced by Subcutaneous and Intratracheal Bleomycin Shows Temporal and Spatial Differences

Intratracheal administration of bleomycin has been reported to cause variable mortality ranging from 8% [14] to 60% [15]; these deaths can be attributed to bleomycin dosing that ranges from 1.0-4.0IU/kg and to the variable potency [16]. Thus we used an optimized dosing of intracheal bleomycin (2.0 IU/kg) that minimizes mouse death but still generates lung fibrosis, and repetitive subcutaneous administration of bleomycin (10 IU/kg) was well tolerated with no mortality (Figure 1). We found that both intratracheal and subcutaneous administration of bleomycin was associated with initial weight loss, which was more pronounced (32% vs 13% by day 10) and sustained in the subcutaneous treatment group (Figure 2). Moreover, changes in general appearance of the mice were visually apparent by day 14 in the subcutaneous, but not in the intratracheally, treated mice (data not shown). Mice in the subcutaneous group appeared disheveled with hunched postures and scruffy coats, in contrast to the sleek-appearing mice with glossy coats in the intratracheal group.

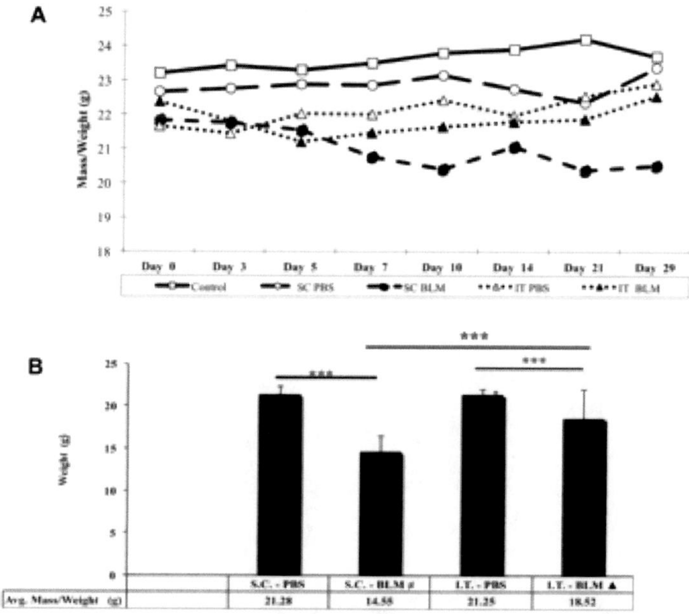

Figure 2. Gross phenotypic changes in mice during experimental protocol. Body mass changes in mice during experimental protocol (A and B). While all mice treated with intratracheal bleomycin loss weight initially, weight loss persisted in the subcutaneously bleomycin-treated mice through day twenty-eight, compared to intratracheally bleomycin-treated mice, whose weight normalized by the end of four weeks (A). At three weeks, mice treated with subcutaneous bleomycin had lost the most weight (B) and weighed, corresponding, the least (A). *** $p < 0.01$.

Histologic Changes in the Lungs

Intratracheal bleomycin has been reported to cause fibrosis by day 14 with maximal fibrotic response extending through days 21-28 [7, 17]. At 28 days of bleomycin given either intratracheally or subcutaneously, patchy lung injury was noted, with areas of the lung appearing relatively normal while other areas showed extensive injury and fibrosis (Figure 3). Subcutaneous bleomycin induced pulmonary changes that were most pronounced at the periphery (Figure 3, solid arrowhead) and around blood vessels (Figure 4, open arrow). Prominent perivascular clusters of spindle-shaped cells suggestive of myofibroblasts and inflammatory infiltrates dominated by foamy histiocytes and lymphocytes were seen (Figure 3). In contrast, mice given intratracheal bleomycin developed injury that was both bronchiolocentric (Figure 4, closed arrow) and vasculocentric (Figure 4, open arrow) with subpleural changes; extensive bronchiolization (Figure 5, closed arrow) was present in areas of injury and fibrosis. Spindle-shaped cells as well as inflammatory cell infiltration consisting of foamy histiocytes and lymphocytes were prominent in the interstitial space.

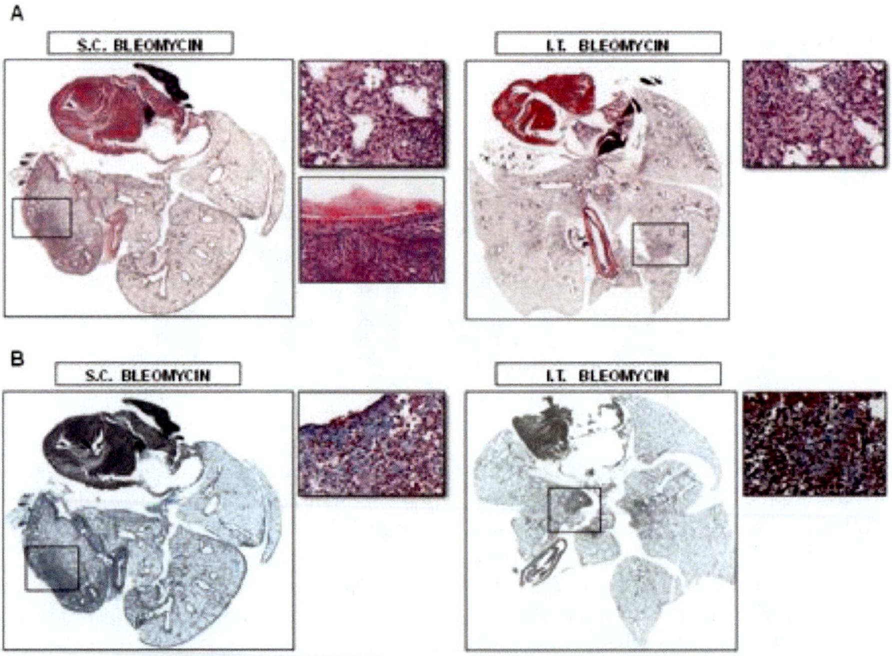

Figure 3. Pulmonary fibrosis is induced by both intratracheal and subcutaneous bleomycin. C57B/L6 mice were given a single dose of intratracheal (IT) bleomycin (BLM), or daily subcutaneous (SC) injections of bleomycin for 14 days, or were left untreated in parallel. At day 28, mice were sacrificed and lungs were processed for analysis. Stereoscopic virtual slice composite images. A. Hematoxylin and eosin (2.5x magnification) B. Masson's Trichrome (2.5x magnification). Untreated mice served as controls.

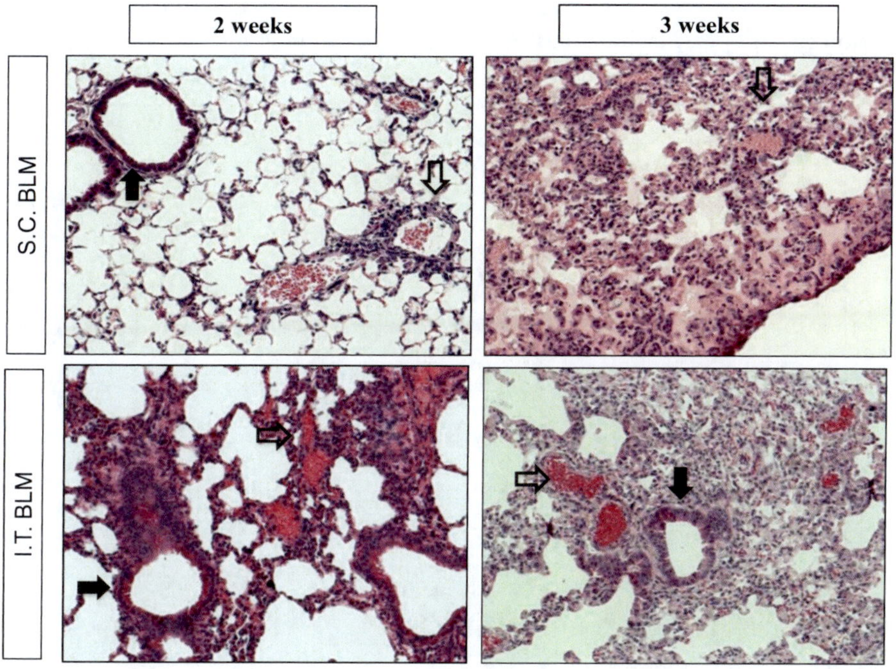

Figure 4. Comparison of lung airways and vasculature between subcutaneous and intratracheal administration of bleomycin at two and three weeks. Open arrow indicates perivascular injury; closed arrow indicates injury around bronchiole.

The pulmonary changes induced by subcutaneous and intratracheal bleomycin showed distinct temporal evolution (Figure 5). At one week, lungs from mice treated with subcutaneous bleomycin showed modest changes with slight cellular infiltration into the interstitium, whereas intratracheal bleomycin caused a robust inflammatory response resulting in dense patches of cellular infiltrates around the airways, in the interstitium, and perivascular regions. At later time points (two to four weeks), both subcutaneous and intratracheal bleomycin models showed patchy pulmonary injury and fibrosis. At two weeks, there was progression of the inflammatory infiltrate into the intersititum and perivascular space in the subcutaneous group, while spindle shaped cells in addition to immune cells were evident in the intratracheal group. At three weeks after subcutaneous bleomycin, the distribution of inflammatory infiltrates was interstitial, pleural/sub-pleural, and strikingly perivascular; there was notably no involvement of the airways. In contrast, three weeks after intratracheal bleomycin treatment, spindle-shaped cells were notably numerous with patchy, dense areas of injury and fibrosis that were peribronchial, perivascular, as well as interstitial in location.

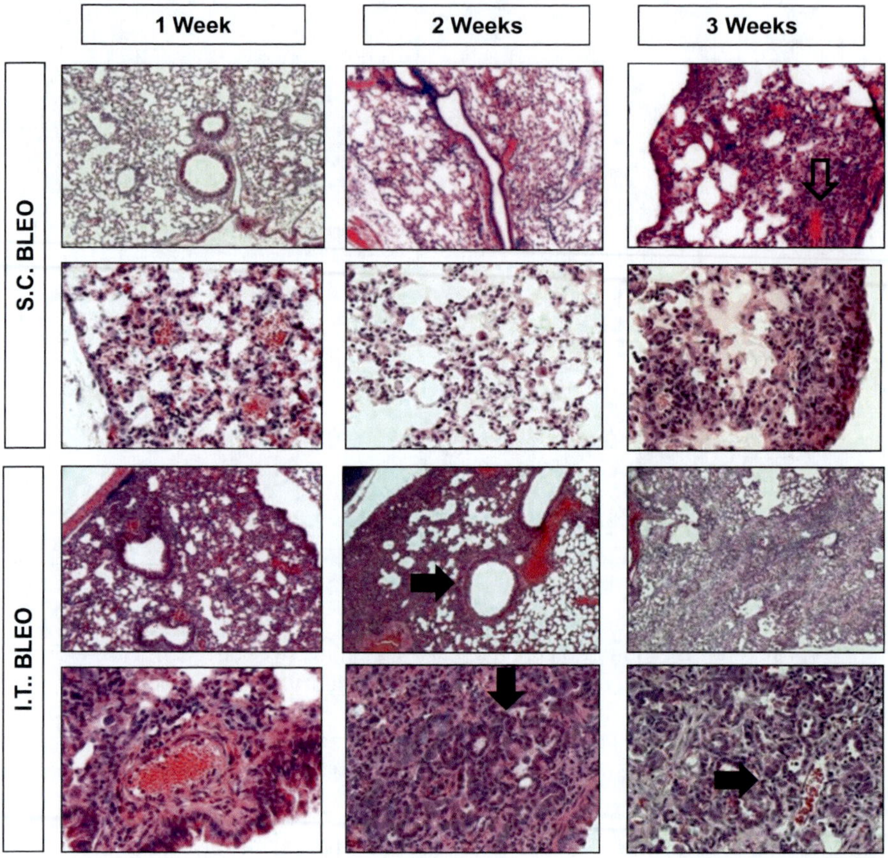

Figure 5. Time-dependent progression of lung fibrosis. Hematoxylin and eosin staining of lungs. Mice treated with bleomycin via subcutaneous (top) or intratracheal (bottom) route were sacrificed at day 7, 14, or 21. Open arrows indicate vascular involvement; closed arrows indicate bronchiolization or involvement of airway.

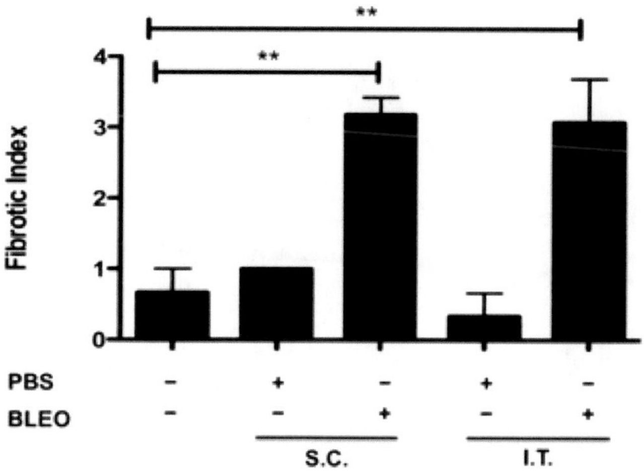

Figure 6. Intensity of lung fibrosis is comparable after administration of subcutaneous and intratracheal bleomycin. Severity of lung fibrosis at day 28 was determined using Ashcroft Index by two independent observers. Results are expressed as the mean ± SD from 3-5 mice per experimental group. **p < 0.01 compared to control and PBS-treated animals.

Previous studies had reported the onset of spontaneous resolution of fibrosis after day 21 in mice treated with intratracheal bleomycin [14, 18]. In the present study, however, Ashcroft scoring [19] revealed that comparable severity of fibrosis persisted at four weeks in both subcutaneous and intratracheal administration of bleomycin (Figure 6). These results were corroborated using the Hubner scoring method, which is a modified method for mouse histopathology [20] (data not shown). The time course of the resolution of fibrosis beyond day 28 was not examined in this study. Significant contrasts in the involvement of the pulmonary vasculature and airways highlighted key differences between the two treatment groups. Subcutaneous bleomycin was associated with prominent early perivascular injury (Figure 4, open arrow, and Figure 5, open arrow). Injury commonly obliterated the small vessels, while largely sparing the nearby airways (Figure 4, closed arrow). In marked contrast, intratracheal administration was associated with a predominantly bronchiolocentric pattern of injury, in which the fibrosis was focused around the small airways and terminal airway ducts (Figure 4 and Figure 5, closed arrows).

Bleomycin-induced experimental pulmonary fibrosis is mediated in part by TGF-β [21-23]. Therefore, we compared phospho-Smad expression as a marker of TGF-β signaling in the lungs from mice given subcutaneous versus intratracheal bleomycin. At week 4, immunostaining showed greater increase in phospho-Smad 2/3 levels in the lungs from subcutaneous bleomycin-treated mice compared to those given intratracheal bleomycin (Figure 7). Correspondingly, levels of total TGF-β in the BAL fluid showed a maximal (3-fold) elevation in mice treated with subcutaneous bleomycin at 3 weeks, whereas in mice given intratracheal bleomycin maximal (3-fold) increase in TGF-β was seen at 2 weeks (Figure 7). These findings suggested that activation of lung TGF-β signaling peaked earlier after intratracheal administration of bleomycin and correlated with the temporal trends of lung injury and fibrosis seen on histology (Figure 5).

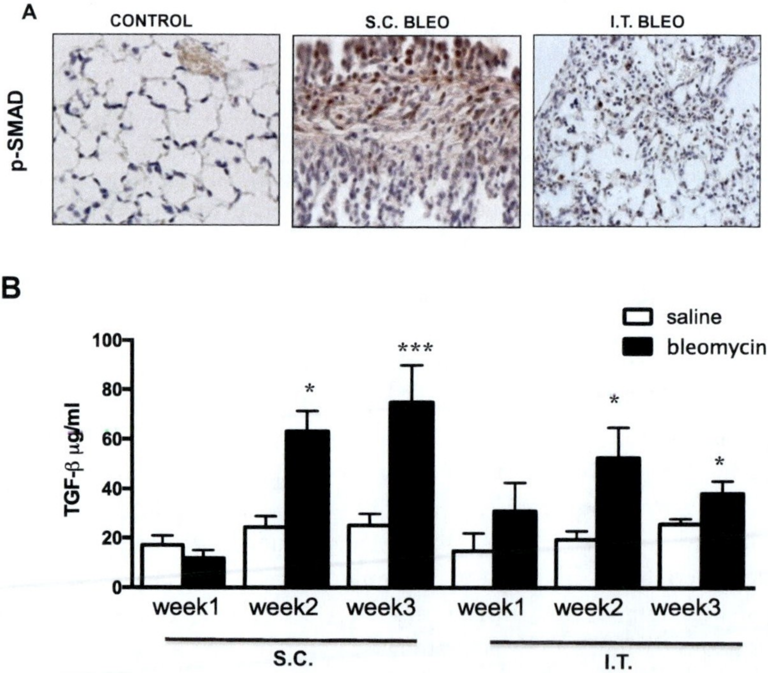

Figure 7. Enhanced TGF-β signaling in the lung. Lungs harvested at week 4 were immunostained with antibodies against phospho-Smad 2/3 (A). Representative images are shown. Bronchoalveolar lavage fluid samples were obtained at the indicated time points. Levels of total TGF-β levels in bronchoalveolar fluid were determined (B). Results are mean ± SD from 7 mice per experimental group. *$p < 0.05$, ***$p < 0.001$ compared to PBS controls.

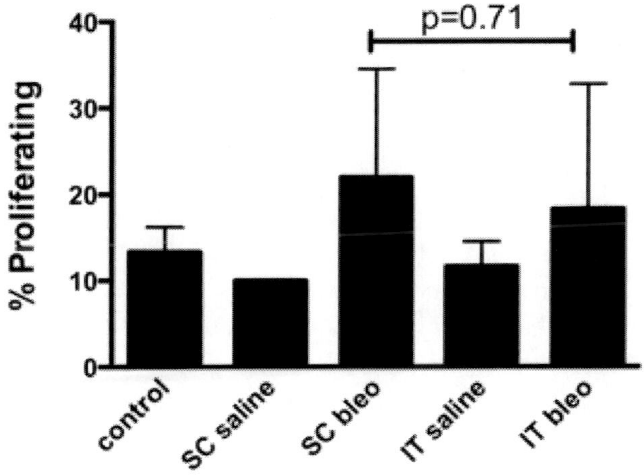

Figure 8. Ki-67 immunostaining of lungs. Increased proliferation demonstrated by enhanced Ki-67 expression in the subcutaneous compared to intratracheal bleomycin induced lung fibrosis model at week 4. The results are expressed as the mean average ± SD values of each experimental group. N = 3-5 animals per group.

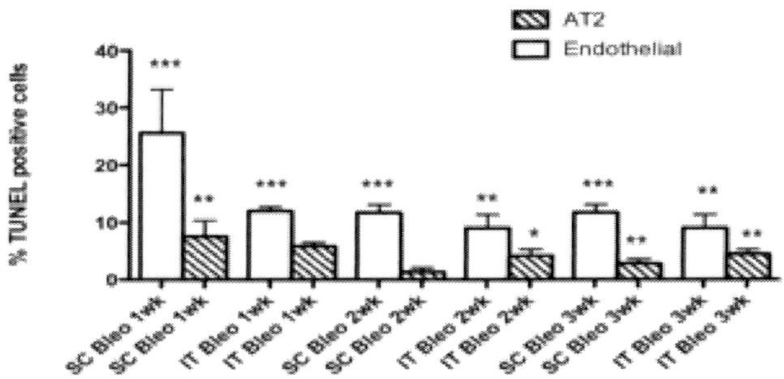

Figure 9. Treatment with either intratracheal or subcutaneous bleomycin increases TUNEL positive endothelial and AT2 cells at all time points. However, there are no statistically significant differences between subcutaneous or intratracheal delivery methods at weeks 1, 2 or 3. N = 7-9 animals per condition. *P < 0.05, **P < 0.01, ***P < 0.001, compared to saline controls (data not shown).

To compare the effects of intratracheal versus subcutaneous bleomycin on lung cell proliferation, Ki-67 staining was performed. Subcutaneous and intratracheal bleomycin induced a comparable increase in pulmonary expression of Ki-67 at week 4 (Figure 8). However, while Ki-67 positivity after subcutaneous bleomycin was localized to intralesional pneumocytes and macrophages, blood vessels, alveolar type 2-like cells, and only rarely to large airways, intratracheal bleomycin resulted in Ki-67 staining that was notably within terminal airways, injured/fibrotic lesions, and lymphoid aggregates (data not shown). Based on our observations regarding the differential nature of the injury (ie peribronchiolar versus perivascular) in the intratracheal versus subcutaneous models, respectively, we speculated that initial pulmonary cell injury and cell death may also be topographically distinct in the two models of fibrosis. To compare the pattern of cell death induced by bleomycin in the two models, TUNEL staining of the lung tissue was performed (Figure 9). At four weeks, following the initial bleomycin injury, the number of TUNEL positive cells in the lungs was markedly elevated in the subcutaneous bleomycin-treated mice compared to mice given intratracheal bleomycin (Figure 10). Notably, apoptosis was seen predominantly in endothelial cells, whereas this was infrequently seen in the intratracheal bleomycin group (Figure 10).

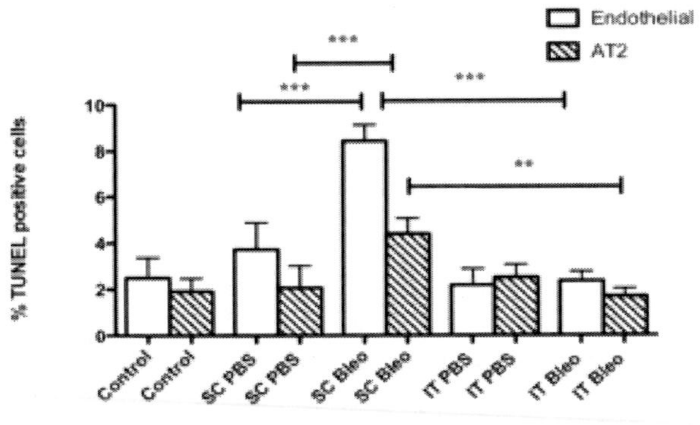

Figure 10. Bleomycin induces apoptosis in lungs. Lungs harvested at day 28 were co-stained with TUNEL as well as markers for AT2 and endothelial cells (SPC and vWF, respectively). Representative images of TUNEL staining was quantified by scoring 100 cells (AT2-positive or endothelial-positive) per high power field and then assessing the number of TUNEL positive cells in each group. Results are expressed as mean $\pm$ SD percentage of TUNEL-positive cells from 5-7 mice/ experimental group. $^{**}p < 0.01$.

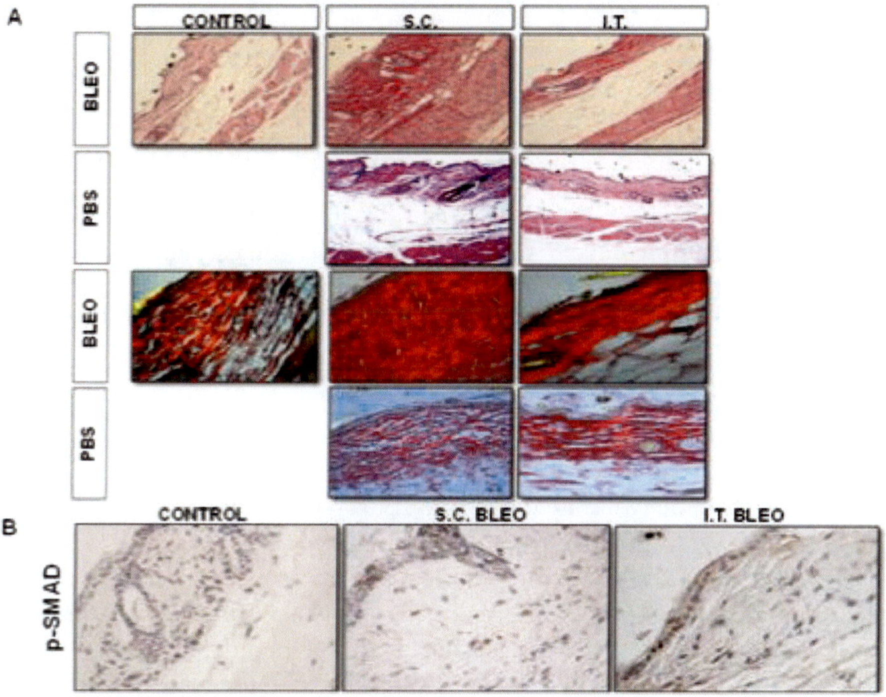

Figure 11. Skin changes induced by bleomycin. Hematoxylin and eosin and Sirius Red staining of skin at week 4 after administration of bleomycin (A). Immunostaining of skin for pSmad 2/3 at week 4 after bleomycin administration (B).

Cutaneous Changes

As bleomycin can cause fibrosis in the skin as well as lung, we wondered whether there were any cutaneous changes associated with the intratracheal administration of bleomycin; therefore skin was harvested from the interscapular region on day 28 [24]. Subcutaneous administration of bleomycin resulted in substantial localized dermal fibrosis, as expected (Figure 11). The dermis showed thickened and sclerotic collagen bundles, accompanied by a loss of intradermal adipose tissue. Skin at locations distant from the site of injection showed no histological alterations (data not shown). Remarkably, skin from mice that received intratracheal bleomycin demonstrated dermal thickening and loss of subcutaneous adipose that was comparable to the lesional skin from subcutaneous injected mice (Figure 6). Morever, increased collagen deposition in the dermis was demonstrated by

Sirius red staining (Figure 11). The number of phospho-Smad positive dermal cells was also elevated compared to skin from PBS-treated and untreated control mice (Figure 11). These findings indicate that intratracheal administration of bleomycin causes skin fibrosis which is histologically indistinguishable from that induced locally by subcutaneous bleomycin. The results suggest that there may be either a systemic response to bleomycin, which causes fibrosis in organs distant to the initial site of injury, or, alternatively, that bleomycin absorbed from the lungs into the systemic circulation is sufficient to initiate a fibrotic response to intratracheal bleomycin in a distant organ.

DISCUSSION

Pulmonary toxicity has long been observed with bleomycin administration [25-27], since its original description by Umezawa et al. in 1966 [28]. It has been suggested that relatively low levels of the inactivating enzyme, bleomycin hydrolase, makes the lung particularly susceptible to the adverse effects of bleomycin [29]. Taking advantage of this finding, the murine model of pulmonary fibrosis induced by systemic (intraperitoneal) bleomycin administration was first described by Adamson et al. [30]. Subsequent studies described the development of delayed pulmonary fibrosis in mice given subcutaneous bleomycin [31, 32].

In the present study, we demonstrate that subcutaneous and intratracheal routes of bleomycin delivery are associated with distinct patterns of lung injury and fibrosis. We found that subcutaneous administration of bleomycin leads to somewhat delayed (starting at two weeks) development of fibrosis with lesions around blood vessels and prominent inflammatory cell infiltration. In contrast, intratracheal administration of bleomycin causes an early inflammatory response that is notable by one week, and fibrotic changes that were most prominent around the airways. In both models, overall cell proliferation is increased after the administration of bleomycin. However, after 4 weeks, cell death, particularly of endothelial cells, was more prominent with subcutaneous bleomycin. Surprisingly, we noted that intratracheal bleomycin delivery was associated with skin changes characterized by dermal fibrosis and enhanced phospho-Smad2/3 expression. This finding cannot be attributed to local manipulation of the skin, as mice treated with saline did not demonstrate these skin changes.

Subcutaneous administration of bleomycin results in systemic effects that may be due to the uptake of bleomycin into the circulation. Kinetic studies have shown that upon subcutaneous injection, bleomycin levels in the lung after three hours were >50% lower compared to the levels following intravenous administration [33]. Fibrotic changes in the lung in the subcutaneous bleomycin model are notably localized to small blood vessels. Repetitive subcutaneous administration of bleomycin presumably causes recurrent vascular-mediated lung injury that leads to the development of pulmonary fibrosis. How bleomycin-induced vascular injury leads to pulmonary fibrosis is unclear, but emerging data suggest that there may be a contribution of fibroblasts from the endothelial compartment via endothelial-mesenchymal transition [34]. Data in other organs using various models of fibrosis also implicate a contribution from the endothelial cells to fibrogenesis [35-37].

Both idiopathic pulmonary fibrosis (IPF) and Systemic Sclerosis-associated Interstitial Lung Disease (SSc-ILD) are associated with significant morbidity and mortality [38, 39]. IPF affects older patients, typically occurring in the sixth and seventh decades, who are more likely to be male, white, and smokers [38], while patients with systemic sclerosis are predominantly female, younger, and African-American [1, 2]. On surgical lung biopsy, histopathology features of IPF include patchy areas of fibrosis and honeycomb changes alternating with normal parenchyma, mild inflammation, and fibroblastic foci [38]; this pattern is referred to as usual interstitial pneumonia (UIP). In contrast, a mixed pattern of fibrosis and inflammation is seen in SSc-ILD; 77% of patients with SSc-ILD have a histologic pattern called non-specific interstitial pneumonia (NSIP), although some patients may have UIP pattern on lung biopsy [40, 41]. The natural history of IPF is believed to be progressive with median survival time of 2-3 year from time of diagnosis, based on retrospective data; more recent studies suggest that the majority of patients develop slowly progressive disease over many years with some patients having an accelerated course [38]. Patients with idiopathic NSIP have markedly better prognosis than those with IPF [42]. In contrast, death from respiratory failure early in the disease course is uncommon in SSc-ILD; unlike the idiopathic forms, survival of SSc-ILD patients with UIP or NSIP patterns does not differ [40, 41].

Despite the dramatic differences in their clinical presentation, pathologic features, and natural history, shared pathways in the pathogenesis of both forms of pulmonary fibrosis have been suggested (reviewed by [1, 2]). Thus research efforts to better understand fibrogenesis for both diseases have focused heavily on *in vivo* murine models using bleomycin. While subcutaneous and intratracheal routes of bleomycin administration both cause pulmonary fibrosis, our results demonstrate that the type of fibrosis is not identical in the two models. We find that intratracheal bleomycin causes bronchiolocentric injury and fibrosis that appears to more closely reflect epithelial injury and activation that are hallmarks of the pathogenesis of IPF [43], the vascular-focused lung injury seen in the subcutaneous bleomycin model may better mimic the pathologic picture of SSc-ILD [1, 44]. The pathogenesis of SSc-ILD is believed to be due to the complex interactions of endothelial cells, leukocytes, and fibroblasts and abnormal vasculature [40]. While fibrosis in both bleomycin administration models shows spontaneous resolution [9], these models continue to be widely used for investigating the acute processes of pulmonary fibrogenesis. Recognition of the critical temporal and spatial differences between the subcutaneous and intratracheal models of bleomycin-induced pulmonary fibrosis will lead to insights regarding the differential contributions of the vascular and airways compartments in lung injury and fibrosis. Our findings will enable investigators to better utilize these two bleomycin models in order to further our understanding of the fundamental processes underlying the complicated disease of pulmonary fibrosis.

MATERIALS AND METHODS

Animals and Experimental Protocols

Eight to twelve week old female C57BL/6J mice with isogenic background (Jackson Labs, Bar Harbor, ME) were provided with Rodent Diet (Harlan, Madison, WI) and water ad lib. Experiments were performed according to institutionally approved protocols and in compliance with the animal welfare guidelines of the Northwestern University Animal Care and Use Committee. In the subcutaneous (SC) model, mice were administered 200 μg/day (approximately 0.2 IU/day or 10 IU/kg) of bleomycin (Mayne Pharma-Hospira, Paramus, NJ) or PBS by subcutaneous injections daily for fourteen days, followed by a fourteen day recovery period prior to sacrifice. In the intratracheal (IT) bleomycin model, a single 50μl injection of PBS or bleomycin 0.04 IU (approximately 40 μg) total in a 20g mouse (2.0 IU/kg) was administered by direct intratracheal instillation into an angiocath using a Hamilton syringe [45]. Mice were sacrificed twenty-eight days after the first subcutaneous injection or intratracheal instillation. For evaluation of the lungs, a 20-gauge angiocatheter was sutured into the trachea. Bronchoalveolar lavage (BAL) was performed by instilling 0.8 ml of sterile PBS into the lungs via angiocatheter and gently aspirating the lavaged fluid; samples were gently spun to remove cells. Then the lungs were removed with the heart *en bloc*, inflated with 4% paraformaldehyde and embedded in paraffin for further analysis.

Histopathologic Evaluation of Lung and Skin

Upon removal, lungs were inflated to 25 cm H2O and fixed in 10% neutrally buffered formalin (NBF) (Fischer Scientific) for 24-36 hours. Skin punch biopsies were fixed for 96 hours in 10% NBF. Tissues were processed through a series of graded alcohols, embedded in paraffin, and serial 4-μm sections were stained with hematoxylin and eosin (H&E, Sigma-Aldrich, St. Louis, MO), Masson's Trichrome (IMEB, San Marcos, CA), Picrosirius Red (Sigma-Aldrich), and Movat's Pentachrome (Rawley Biochemical, Danvers, MA). Stained tissue slides were visualized and photographed using a Nikon Ellipse 80i microscope (Software: NIS – Elements D 2.30) (Huntley, Il), under coherent light or with a polarized filter at 100x and 400x magnifications. Stereoscopic virtual images of whole lungs were photographed using a Zeiss Axioskope (Zeiss, Oberkochen, Germany) using Neurolucida Software at 2.5x magnification. Images were obtained by digital capture.

Immunohistochemistry

Four-μm sections of lesional skin and lungs were deparaffinized, rehydrated, and immersed in TBS-T buffer (Tris-buffered saline and 0.1% Tween 20), then treated with target retrieval solution (DAKO, Carpinteria, CA) at 95°C for 10 minutes prior to incubation with primary antibodies against α-smooth muscle actin (1:750x dilution) (Sigma-Aldridge, St. Louis, MO), phospho-Smad2/3 (1:150x dilution) (from Santa Cruz Biotechnology, Santa Cruz, CA), and Ki-67 (1:100x dilution) (Dako). Substitution of the primary antibody with isotype IgG (Dako) served as negative controls. Sections were counterstained with hematoxylin, mounted with Histomount (ThermoFisher Scientific), and photographed using a Nikon Ellipse 80i microscope (Software NIS – Elements D 2.30, Huntley, Il) at 100x or 400x magnification under coherent light. Images were obtained by digital capture. Stained lung sections were scored using rodent modified Ashcroft's [19] and Hubner's methods [20] independently by two experienced lung pathologists who were blinded to the experimental conditions.

Bronchoalveolar Fluid TGF-β Content

After placement of an angiocatheter into the trachea, 0.8ml of sterile saline was lavaged into the lungs and aspirated back. The samples were gently spun at 1,000x*g* for 10 minutes to remove cells. TGF-β immunoassay was performed following the manufacturer's protocol (R&D Systems, Minneapolis, MN) as previously described [46].

TUNEL Staining

Cell death in the lungs was assessed by the TUNEL *in situ* cell death detection kit (Roche Diagnostics) according to the manufacturer's instructions [47]. Formalin-fixed, paraffin-embedded lung sections were analyzed by immunohistochemistry using antibodies for von Willebrand factor (VWF, A0082, DAKO) and α-SMA (ab7817, Abcam), as previously described [48].

Statistical Analysis

Statistical analysis was performed by Student's t test or one-way analysis of variance (ANOVA) followed by Bonferoni's multiple comparison test. A p value < 0.05 was considered significant. Statistical calculations were performed using GraphPad Prism software (Graph Pad Software Inc, La Jolla, CA).

Competing Interests: none.

Authors' Contributions: APL, ELH, DM, and JV conceived and designed the experiments; APL, ELH, DM, JS, YG, KR, RH, and AY performed the experiments and analyzed the data; APL and JV wrote the manuscript.

Grant Support: K08HL093216 and P30HL101292 to A. P. L., DOD W81XWH-12-1-0471 to J.V.

REFERENCES

[1] Murray LA, Rubinowitz A, Herzog EL. Interstitial lung disease: is interstitial lung disease the same as scleroderma lung disease? *Current opinion in rheumatology.* 2012; 24(6):656-62. doi: 10.1097/BOR. 0b013e3283588de4. PubMed PMID: 22955020.

[2] Herzog EL, Mathur A, Tager AM, Feghali-Bostwick C, Schneider F, Varga J. Review: interstitial lung disease associated with systemic sclerosis and idiopathic pulmonary fibrosis: how similar and distinct? *Arthritis and rheumatology.* 2014;66(8):1967-78. doi: 10.1002/art.38702. PubMed PMID: 24838199; PubMed Central PMCID: PMC4340472.

[3] Selman M, King TE, Pardo A. Idiopathic pulmonary fibrosis: prevailing and evolving hypotheses about its pathogenesis and implications for therapy. *Ann Intern Med.* 2001;134(2):136-51. PubMed PMID: 11177318.

[4] Noble PW, Barkauskas CE, Jiang D. Pulmonary fibrosis: patterns and perpetrators. *The Journal of clinical investigation.* 2012;122(8):2756-62. doi: 10.1172/JCI60323. PubMed PMID: 22850886; PubMed Central PMCID: PMC3408732.

[5] Fischer A, du Bois R. Interstitial lung disease in connective tissue disorders. *Lancet.* 2012;380(9842):689-98. doi: 10.1016/S0140-6736(12)61079-4. PubMed PMID: 22901890.

[6] Baron RM, Choi AJ, Owen CA, Choi AM. Genetically manipulated mouse models of lung disease: potential and pitfalls. American journal of physiology *Lung cellular and molecular physiology.* 2012;302(6): L485-97. doi: 10.1152/ajplung.00085.2011. PubMed PMID: 22198907; PubMed Central PMCID: PMC4074003.

[7] Moore BB, Hogaboam CM. Murine models of pulmonary fibrosis. *American journal of physiology Lung cellular and molecular physiology.* 2008;294(2):L152-60. PubMed PMID: 17993587.

[8] Moeller A, Ask K, Warburton D, Gauldie J, Kolb M. The bleomycin animal model: a useful tool to investigate treatment options for idiopathic pulmonary fibrosis? *Int J Biochem Cell Biol.* 2008;40(3):362-82. doi: 10.1016/j.biocel.2007.08.011. PubMed PMID: 17936056; PubMed Central PMCID: PMC2323681.

[9] Mouratis MA, Aidinis V. Modeling pulmonary fibrosis with bleomycin. *Current opinion in pulmonary medicine.* 2011;17(5):355-61. doi: 10.1097/MCP.0b013e328349ac2b. PubMed PMID: 21832918.

[10] Dees C, Schlottmann I, Funke R, Distler A, Palumbo-Zerr K, Zerr P, Lin NY, Beyer C, Distler O, Schett G, Distler JH. The Wnt antagonists DKK1 and SFRP1 are downregulated by promoter hypermethylation in systemic sclerosis. *Ann Rheum Dis.* 2014;73(6):1232-9. doi: 10.1136/annrheumdis-2012-203194. PubMed PMID: 23698475.

[11] Ozgen M, Koca SS, Dagli AF, Gundogdu B, Ustundag B, Isik A. Mycophenolate mofetil and daclizumab targeting T lymphocytes in bleomycin-induced experimental scleroderma. *Clinical and experimental dermatology.* 2012;37(1):48-54. doi: 10.1111/j.1365-2230.2011.04201.x. PubMed PMID: 22182434.

[12] Wei J, Melichian D, Komura K, Hinchcliff M, Lam AP, Lafyatis R, Gottardi CJ, MacDougald OA, Varga J. Canonical Wnt signaling induces skin fibrosis and subcutaneous lipoatrophy: a novel mouse model for scleroderma? *Arthritis Rheum.* 2011;63(6):1707-17. doi: 10.1002/art.30312. PubMed PMID: 21370225; PubMed Central PMCID: PMC3124699.

[13] Balistreri E, Garcia-Gonzalez E, Selvi E, Akhmetshina A, Palumbo K, Lorenzini S, Maggio R, Lucattelli M, Galeazzi M, Distler JW. The cannabinoid WIN55, 212-2 abrogates dermal fibrosis in scleroderma bleomycin model. *Ann Rheum Dis.* 2011;70(4):695-9. doi: 10.1136/ard.2010.137539. PubMed PMID: 21177293.

[14] Degryse AL, Tanjore H, Xu XC, Polosukhin VV, Jones BR, McMahon FB, Gleaves LA, Blackwell TS, Lawson WE. Repetitive Intratracheal Bleomycin Models Several Features of Idiopathic Pulmonary Fibrosis. *American journal of physiology Lung cellular and molecular physiology.* 2010. Epub 2010/06/22. doi: ajplung.00026.2010 [pii] 10.1152/ajplung.00026.2010. PubMed PMID: 20562227.

[15] Henderson WR, Jr., Chi EY, Ye X, Nguyen C, Tien YT, Zhou B, Borok Z, Knight DA, Kahn M. Inhibition of Wnt/beta-catenin/CREB binding protein (CBP) signaling reverses pulmonary fibrosis. *Proc Natl Acad Sci*

U S A. 2010;107(32):14309-14. Epub 2010/07/28. doi: 1001520107 [pii] 10.1073/pnas.1001520107. PubMed PMID: 20660310.

[16] Stefanou A, Siderov J, Society of Hospital Pharmacists of Australia Committee of Specialty Practice in O. Medical errors. Dosage nomenclature of bleomycin needs to be standardised to avoid errors. *Bmj*. 2001;322(7299):1423-4. PubMed PMID: 11417551.

[17] Peng R, Sridhar S, Tyagi G, Phillips JE, Garrido R, Harris P, Burns L, Renteria L, Woods J, Chen L, Allard J, Ravindran P, Bitter H, Liang Z, Hogaboam CM, Kitson C, Budd DC, Fine JS, Bauer CM, Stevenson CS. Bleomycin induces molecular changes directly relevant to idiopathic pulmonary fibrosis: a model for "active" disease. *PLoS One*. 2013;8(4):e59348. doi: 10.1371/journal.pone.0059348. PubMed PMID: 23565148; PubMed Central PMCID: PMC3614979.

[18] Chung MP, Monick MM, Hamzeh NY, Butler NS, Powers LS, Hunninghake GW. Role of repeated lung injury and genetic background in bleomycin-induced fibrosis. *Am J Respir Cell Mol Biol*. 2003;29(3 Pt 1):375-80. doi: 10.1165/rcmb.2003-0029OC. PubMed PMID: 12676806.

[19] Ashcroft T, Simpson JM, Timbrell V. Simple method of estimating severity of pulmonary fibrosis on a numerical scale. *Journal of clinical pathology*. 1988;41(4):467-70. PubMed PMID: 3366935; PubMed Central PMCID: PMC1141479.

[20] Hubner RH, Gitter W, El Mokhtari NE, Mathiak M, Both M, Bolte H, Freitag-Wolf S, Bewig B. Standardized quantification of pulmonary fibrosis in histological samples. *BioTechniques*. 2008;44(4):507-11, 14-7. doi: 10.2144/000112729. PubMed PMID: 18476815.

[21] Westergren-Thorsson G, Hernnas J, Sarnstrand B, Oldberg A, Heinegard D, Malmstrom A. Altered expression of small proteoglycans, collagen, and transforming growth factor-beta 1 in developing bleomycin-induced pulmonary fibrosis in rats. *The Journal of clinical investigation*. 1993;92(2):632-7. doi: 10.1172/JCI116631. PubMed PMID: 7688761; PubMed Central PMCID: PMC294895.

[22] King SL, Lichtler AC, Rowe DW, Xie R, Long GL, Absher MP, Cutroneo KR. Bleomycin stimulates pro-alpha 1 (I) collagen promoter through transforming growth factor beta response element by intracellular and extracellular signaling. *The Journal of biological chemistry*. 1994;269(18):13156-61. PubMed PMID: 7513699.

[23] Kolb M, Margetts PJ, Galt T, Sime PJ, Xing Z, Schmidt M, Gauldie J. Transient transgene expression of decorin in the lung reduces the fibrotic response to bleomycin. *Am J Respir Crit Care Med.* 2001;163(3 Pt 1): 770-7. doi: 10.1164/ajrccm.163.3.2006084. PubMed PMID: 11254537.

[24] Bhattacharyya S, Kelley K, Melichian DS, Tamaki Z, Fang F, Su Y, Feng G, Pope RM, Budinger GR, Mutlu GM, Lafyatis R, Radstake T, Feghali-Bostwick C, Varga J. Toll-like receptor 4 signaling augments transforming growth factor-beta responses: a novel mechanism for maintaining and amplifying fibrosis in scleroderma. *Am J Pathol.* 2013;182(1):192-205. doi: 10.1016/j.ajpath.2012.09.007. PubMed PMID: 23141927; PubMed Central PMCID: PMC3538029.

[25] Rudders RA, Hensley GT. Bleomycin pulmonary toxicity. Chest. 1973;63(4):627-8. PubMed PMID: 4121121.

[26] Bedrossian CW, Luna MA, Mackay B, Lichtiger B. Ultrastructure of pulmonary bleomycin toxicity. *Cancer.* 1973;32(1):44-51. PubMed PMID: 4123792.

[27] Krous HF, Hamlin WB. Pulmonary toxicity due to bleomycin. Report of a case. *Archives of pathology.* 1973;95(6):407-10. PubMed PMID: 4121790.

[28] Umezawa H, Maeda K, Takeuchi T, Okami Y. New antibiotics, bleomycin A and B. *The Journal of antibiotics.* 1966;19(5):200-9. PubMed PMID: 5953301.

[29] Sebti SM, Mignano JE, Jani JP, Srimatkandada S, Lazo JS. Bleomycin hydrolase: molecular cloning, sequencing, and biochemical studies reveal membership in the cysteine proteinase family. *Biochemistry.* 1989;28(16):6544-8. PubMed PMID: 2477059.

[30] Adamson IY, Bowden DH. The pathogenesis of bleomycin-induced pulmonary fibrosis in mice. *Am J Pathol.* 1974;77(2):185-97. PubMed PMID: 4141224; PubMed Central PMCID: PMC1910906.

[31] Sikic BI, Young DM, Mimnaugh EG, Gram TE. Quantification of bleomycin pulmonary toxicity in mice by changes in lung hydroxyproline content and morphometric histopathology. *Cancer research.* 1978;38(3):787-92. PubMed PMID: 75060.

[32] Yamamoto T, Takagawa S, Katayama I, Yamazaki K, Hamazaki Y, Shinkai H, Nishioka K. Animal model of sclerotic skin. I: Local injections of bleomycin induce sclerotic skin mimicking scleroderma. *The Journal of investigative dermatology.* 1999;112(4):456-62. doi: 10.1046/j.1523-1747.1999.00528.x. PubMed PMID: 10201529.

[33] Bier J, Benders P, Wenzel M, Bitter K. Kinetics of 57Co-bleomycin in mice after intravenous, subcutaneous and intratumoral injection. *Cancer.* 1979;44(4):1194-200. PubMed PMID: 91421.

[34] Hashimoto N, Phan SH, Imaizumi K, Matsuo M, Nakashima H, Kawabe T, Shimokata K, Hasegawa Y. Endothelial-mesenchymal transition in bleomycin-induced pulmonary fibrosis. *Am J Respir Cell Mol Biol.* 2010;43(2):161-72. doi: 10.1165/rcmb.2009-0031OC. PubMed PMID: 19767450; PubMed Central PMCID: PMC2937229.

[35] Zeisberg EM, Potenta SE, Sugimoto H, Zeisberg M, Kalluri R. Fibroblasts in kidney fibrosis emerge via endothelial-to-mesenchymal transition. *J Am Soc Nephrol.* 2008;19(12):2282-7. doi: 10.1681/ASN. 2008050513. PubMed PMID: 18987304; PubMed Central PMCID: PMC2588112.

[36] Kitao A, Sato Y, Sawada-Kitamura S, Harada K, Sasaki M, Morikawa H, Shiomi S, Honda M, Matsui O, Nakanuma Y. Endothelial to mesenchymal transition via transforming growth factor-beta1/Smad activation is associated with portal venous stenosis in idiopathic portal hypertension. *Am J Pathol.* 2009;175(2):616-26. doi: 10.2353/ ajpath.2009.081061. PubMed PMID: 19608867; PubMed Central PMCID: PMC2716961.

[37] Leach HG, Chrobak I, Han R, Trojanowska M. Endothelial cells recruit macrophages and contribute to a fibrotic milieu in bleomycin lung injury. *Am J Respir Cell Mol Biol.* 2013;49(6):1093-101. doi: 10.1165/rcmb.2013-0152OC. PubMed PMID: 23885794; PubMed Central PMCID: PMC3931119.

[38] Raghu G, Collard HR, Egan JJ, Martinez FJ, Behr J, Brown KK, Colby TV, Cordier JF, Flaherty KR, Lasky JA, Lynch DA, Ryu JH, Swigris JJ, Wells AU, Ancochea J, Bouros D, Carvalho C, Costabel U, Ebina M, Hansell DM, Johkoh T, Kim DS, King TE, Jr., Kondoh Y, Myers J, Muller NL, Nicholson AG, Richeldi L, Selman M, Dudden RF, Griss BS, Protzko SL, Schunemann HJ, Fibrosis AEJACoIP. An official ATS/ERS/JRS/ALAT statement: idiopathic pulmonary fibrosis: evidence-based guidelines for diagnosis and management. *Am J Respir Crit Care Med.* 2011;183(6):788-824. doi: 10.1164/rccm.2009-040GL. PubMed PMID: 21471066.

[39] Bussone G, Mouthon L. Interstitial lung disease in systemic sclerosis. *Autoimmunity reviews*. 2011;10(5):248-55. doi: 10.1016/j.autrev.2010. 09.012. PubMed PMID: 20863911.

[40] Solomon JJ, Olson AL, Fischer A, Bull T, Brown KK, Raghu G. Scleroderma lung disease. *European respiratory review : an official journal of the European Respiratory Society*. 2013;22(127):6-19. doi: 10.1183/09059180.00005512. PubMed PMID: 23457159; PubMed Central PMCID: PMC4103193.

[41] Bouros D, Wells AU, Nicholson AG, Colby TV, Polychronopoulos V, Pantelidis P, Haslam PL, Vassilakis DA, Black CM, du Bois RM. Histopathologic subsets of fibrosing alveolitis in patients with systemic sclerosis and their relationship to outcome. *Am J Respir Crit Care Med.* 2002;165(12):1581-6. PubMed PMID: 12070056.

[42] American Thoracic Society/European Respiratory Society International Multidisciplinary Consensus Classification of the Idiopathic Interstitial Pneumonias. This joint statement of the American Thoracic Society (ATS), and the European Respiratory Society (ERS) was adopted by the ATS board of directors, June 2001 and by the ERS Executive Committee, June 2001. *Am J Respir Crit Care Med.* 2002;165(2):277-304. PubMed PMID: 11790668.

[43] Selman M, Pardo A. Role of epithelial cells in idiopathic pulmonary fibrosis: from innocent targets to serial killers. *Proceedings of the American Thoracic Society*. 2006;3(4):364-72. Epub 2006/06/02. doi: 3/4/364 [pii] 10.1513/pats.200601-003TK. PubMed PMID: 16738202.

[44] Homer RJ, Elias JA, Lee CG, Herzog E. Modern concepts on the role of inflammation in pulmonary fibrosis. *Archives of pathology and laboratory medicine*. 2011;135(6):780-8. doi: 10.1043/2010-0296-RA.1. PubMed PMID: 21631273.

[45] Flozak AS, Lam AP, Russell S, Jain M, Peled ON, Sheppard KA, Beri R, Mutlu GM, Budinger GR, Gottardi CJ. Beta-catenin/T-cell factor signaling is activated during lung injury and promotes the survival and migration of alveolar epithelial cells. *The Journal of biological chemistry*. 2010;285(5):3157-67. Epub 2009/11/26. doi: M109.070326 [pii]10.1074/jbc.M109.070326. PubMed PMID: 19933277; PubMed Central PMCID: PMC2823449.

[46] Mutlu GM, Budinger GR, Wu M, Lam AP, Zirk A, Rivera S, Urich D, Chiarella SE, Go LH, Ghosh AK, Selman M, Pardo A, Varga J, Kamp DW, Chandel NS, Sznajder JI, Jain M. Proteasomal inhibition after injury prevents fibrosis by modulating TGF-beta(1) signalling. *Thorax.* 2012;67(2):139-46. doi: 10.1136/thoraxjnl-2011-200717. PubMed PMID: 21921091; PubMed Central PMCID: PMC3595535.

[47] Murray LA, Chen Q, Kramer MS, Hesson DP, Argentieri RL, Peng X, Gulati M, Homer RJ, Russell T, van Rooijen N, Elias JA, Hogaboam CM, Herzog EL. TGF-beta driven lung fibrosis is macrophage dependent and blocked by Serum amyloid P. *Int J Biochem Cell Biol.* 2011;43(1):154-62. doi: 10.1016/j.biocel.2010.10.013. PubMed PMID: 21044893.

[48] Jakubzick C, Choi ES, Joshi BH, Keane MP, Kunkel SL, Puri RK, Hogaboam CM. Therapeutic attenuation of pulmonary fibrosis via targeting of IL-4- and IL-13-responsive cells. *Journal of immunology.* 2003;171(5):2684-93. PubMed PMID: 12928422.

In: Cystic and Idiopathic Pulmonary Fibrosis ISBN: 978-1-63485-508-2
Editor: Lorenzo Robertson

Chapter 6

SLEEP DISORDERS IN IDIOPATHIC PULMONARY FIBROSIS

Hans Schweisfurth [*]
Institute for Pulmonary Research (IPR),
Cottbus, Germany

ABSTRACT

Idiopathic pulmonary fibrosis (IPF) is the most common idiopathic interstitial disease of the lung of unknown etiology with a median survival time of about 3 years. IPF occurs mainly in men older than 60 years who have comorbidities such as pulmonary hypertension, COPD, lung cancer, gastro-esophageal reflux, ischemic heart disease and obstructive sleep apnoea. IPF affects the quality of life (QL) by fatigue mostly associated with poor sleep quality. In IPF patients alteration in sleep architecture, increased sleep fragmentation and slow wave sleep periods are detectable. During the vulnerable REM sleep stage sleep related hypoventilation and obstructive sleep apnea syndrome are often observed. These sleep disorders in IPF are associated with reduction of QL and increased risk of mortality. Therefore, clinicians should refer patients with IPF to sleep centers for the diagnosis and possible treatment of sleep related disorders with continuous positive airway pressure devices. In the absence of an effective therapy for IPF, the treatment of sleep disorders could significantly improve the QL of these patients.

---

[*] E-Mail: pulfin@t-online.de.

INTRODUCTION

Idiopathic pulmonary fibrosis (IPF) is the most common idiopathic interstitial disease of the lung of unknown etiology, dominated by males, with a median survival time of about 3 years [1, 2, 3].

Identification and treatment of complicating comorbidities such as obstructive sleep apnoea (OSA) may have a significant impact on survival in IPF. OSA is characterized by cessation of regular breathing during sleep. Apnoea means the complete cessation of respiration and hypopnoea is marked by partial or decreased respiration. For the diagnosis of sleep apnoea, each apnoeic or hypopnoeic event must last a minimum of 10 s. Each respiratory event generally results in repeated arousals from sleep as well as nocturnal hypoxemia. OSA is considered as mild if the apnoea hypopnoea index (AHI) is between 5 and 15 events per hour, moderate 15 -30 events per hour, and severe if more than 30 events per hour occur [4].

In healthy subjects, sleep represents a state of restoration covering approximately one-third of human life. Sleep hypoventilation, especially during the vulnerable rapid eye movement (REM) sleep period, is well tolerated by healthy subjects, but may represent a hazardous risk in patients with chronic respiratory diseases [5, 6].

During REM sleep, the diaphragm remains the only active respiratory muscle, while accessory muscles are temporarily not functional.

Research of sleep disorders has mainly focused on patients with chronic obstructive pulmonary disease (COPD). Significant changes in oxygenation or breathing parameters have been described in patients with COPD, particularly during the vulnerable REM sleep period [7, 8].

FEATURES OF SLEEP-RELATED DISORDERS

Although multiple significant oxygen desaturations are characteristic of nocturnal oximetry in patients with sleep apnoea, the physiologic mechanism driving sleep disordered breathing in the presence of pulmonary fibrosis manifests predominantly as hypopnoeas rather than apneic events [9, 10].

Interestingly a recent study showed that pulmonary function parameters such as lung volumes, forced vital capacity or transfer factor do not correlate inversely with the AHI [9].

In patients with OSA, daytime sleepiness as measured by the Epworth Sleepiness Scale is a poor predictor of OSA severity. The observed nocturnal hypoxia almost invariably disrupts sleep architecture and appears to have a greater impact on the quality of life (QL) in these individuals [10, 11].

In a small cohort of patients AHI appeared to correlate positively with body mass index and negatively with the forced expiratory volume in 1 s [12]. The impairment in pulmonary physiology appears to be linked to the interdependence between upper airways in OSA and lung volumes. In snorers with OSA, a decrease in lung volumes results in a dramatic reduction in the pharyngeal cross-sectional area, a phenomenon that is amplified by the fibrotic process which occurs in patients with diffuse parenchymal lung fibrosis. Studies in which the functional residual capacity was increased have shown a subsequent improvement in sleep architecture and improvement in AHI [13, 14].

Recurrent, chronic micro aspiration associated with gastroesophageal reflux disease (GERD) worsens hypoxemia in patients with OSA and IPF. Studies have shown amelioration of GERD when the OSA in these patients is treated with continuous positive airway pressure (CPAP), which could potentially lead to a retardation of disease progression [15].

Reduced sleep quality is present in most patients with IPF and is an important predictor of quality of life [16 - 19]. But some authors did not find any association between IPF and sleep disorders [20].

CLINICAL STUDIES

Sleep-related breathing disorders occur commonly in IPF. This may be attributable to the increased prevalence of nocturnal oxygen desaturations, coughing with arousals, and increased respiratory drive that occur in these individuals. The International Classification of Sleep Disorders (ICSD) categorizes sleep-related breathing disorders in IPF to a separate group termed "sleep disorders with sleep-related hypoventilation and hypoxemia in parenchymal or vascular lung diseases" and the most recent ICSD-3 classification in 2014 placed them in the unique subgroup of "sleep-related hypoxemia disorder "given the distinctive nature of oxygen desaturation that occurs in these individuals [21, 22].

Published studies related to sleep in IPF should be divided into those performed before and after publication of the 2002 American Thoracic Society/European Respiratory Society criteria for the diagnosis of IPF [23].

The studies between1980 and 1990 included small numbers of patients with a variety of restrictive lung diseases. Studies performed after the 2002 guidelines mostly included only patients with a confirmed diagnosis of IPF. This is important, as IPF affects only the lungs, while other interstitial lung diseases may occur in presence of underlying systemic diseases. Recent methodological differences, such as a change in the definition of hypopnoeas as well as more sophisticated devices applied for event detection, also complicates the comparison between older and more recent studies [24].

The nocturnal pulse oximetry of a typical patient with severe IPF usually shows a specific pattern of multiple phasic desaturations which are caused by hypoventilation. This may lead to fragmentation of sleep and impairment of sleep quality [25]. Furthermore, a reduction in REM sleep and an increase in stage 1 sleep have been observed in patients with severe pulmonary fibrosis [12, 26, 27].

In IPF patients daytime PaO2 levels while awake appear to be predictive of the extent of nocturnal oxygen desaturation and presence of OSA during sleep [25].

The majority of IPF patients have an AHI of > 5 events per hour and up to 65% of IPF patients have an AHI of >15 that is consistent with moderate or severe OSA [9, 28, 29]. OSA is more common in IPF than in other fibrotic interstitial lung diseases and its severity correlates with extent of fibrosis and is associated with repetitive injury to the alveolar epithelium and has been proposed as a potential cause of IPF [29 - 32].

Improved QL and sleep quality have been demonstrated in small nonrandomized studies of IPF patients with OSA who are compliant with CPAP treatment [28, 33]. Similar benefits were observed in the subgroup of patients without daytime sleepiness prior to initiation of CPAP [28].

It may therefore be appropriate to screen all IPF patients for sleep-disordered breathing because of the high prevalence of OSA in IPF and the poor sensitivity of clinical features and screening tools such as the Epworth Sleepiness Scale [9, 28]. In regions with limited access to polysomnography, it is likely reasonable to screen for OSA with overnight oximetry, and in patients with suggestive findings the application of CPAP therapy should be initiated [34].

Based on recent literature reporting an increased incidence of OSA in patients with IPF, the most recent IPF guidelines include OSA among IPF-associated comorbidities [35].

Sleep disturbances are likely to play a major role in overall QL as well as in morbidity and mortality in IPF patients (Table 1) [19, 25, 36, 37].

Table 1. Sleep disturbances in patients with IPF [4, 59]

Sleep macro- and micro-architecture:
Increased stage 1 sleep
Decreased REM and slow-wave sleep
Decreased sleep efficiency
Increased WASO
Increased arousal index
Respiratory pattern:
Increased respiratory frequency during sleep
Rapid and shallow breathing (especially during REM sleep)
Nocturnal oxygenation parameters:
Episodic desaturation during REM sleep
Desaturation during non-REM sleep
Desaturation due to respiratory events (apnoeas and hypopnoeas)
Sleep disordered breathing:
Increased incidence of obstructive sleep apnoea
Other sleep problems:
Increased periodic leg movements during sleep
Insomnia
Nocturnal cough and choking
Thirst during the night
Nocturnal diuresis
Impotence
Gastro-esophageal reflux

REM: rapid eye movement; WASO: wake time after sleep onset.

In patients with IPF sleep is found to be markedly disturbed. Most studies agree on the findings of abnormal sleep macro- and micro-architecture, respiratory breathing patterns, and oxygen desaturation with features of hypoventilation, especially during the vulnerable REM period.

The AHI was found to be low even though hypoxemia and obesity were noted in several of these patients. ILD patients had a higher respiratory frequency than controls, during both wakefulness and sleep. Respiratory frequency during sleep showed no significant change in IPF patients in contrast to the noted decrease in the control group. It is hypothesized that the lack of change might be due to the maintenance of reflexes causing rapid, shallow breathing during sleep. The same breathing pattern was observed in a more recent study [38].

The first study reporting the need for a high awareness for OSA in IPF population was a retrospective study in 18 patients with IPF, who had been referred for overnight polysomnography to investigate complaints suggestive of sleep disordered breathing [12].

OSA was confirmed in 11 patients and the rest were diagnosed with upper airway resistance syndrome or primary snoring. The authors pointed out that despite growing awareness of OSA among healthcare providers, treating physicians may defer sleep testing because IPF is characterized by such a rapidly progressive course, leading them to focus on more acute problems such as dyspnoea and limitations in daily activities. Obesity and the magnitude of the pulmonary function test impairment were recognized as predictor factors for OSA. Restrictive pulmonary diseases are characterized by decreased lung volumes that can reduce the upper airway stability and increase the resistance on the upper airway. These changes can facilitate upper airway collapse, especially during REM sleep when functional residual capacity is further reduced due to the inactivity of the intercostal muscles [13, 14, 39].

Another significant finding of this study was the increased frequency of restless-leg syndrome and periodic leg movements during sleep in this population. The first prospective study on the topic OSA in IPF was performed in the USA including 50 IPF patients [9]. OSA was diagnosed in 88% of subjects. 10 (20%) subjects had mild OSA and 34 (68%) had moderate-to-severe OSA. Neither the Epworth Sleepiness Scale nor the Sleep Apnoea Scale of Sleep Disorders Questionnaire, alone or in combination, was a strong screening tool. The study did not demonstrate an inverse relationship between forced vital capacity and AHI, contrary to the previously described theory that decreased lung volumes predispose to OSA by reducing the upper airway stability and increasing resistance due to a decreased traction on the upper airway. The authors claimed that the lack of inverse correlation between the pulmonary function test (PFT) and the severity of sleep apnoea may be explained by the PFT, which was performed in the upright or standing position. PFT in the supine position of the patient may be more accurate at predicting sleep lung volumes, and may better display interdependence between the upper airway and lung volumes during sleep. A limitation of the study was the fact that the included patients were receiving corticosteroids or other treatments for IPF. This was excluded in a multicenter study in which polysomnography was performed in 34 treatment-naïve patients soon after the diagnosis of IPF. 15 (44%) subjects had mild and five (15%) had moderate-to-severe OSA, while 14 (41%) subjects were normal [29].

Based on these studies, the incidence of OSA is high in IPF patients, but it should be regarded that IPF occurs mostly in those over the age of 60 years, an age where OSA increases even among the normal population. Data from the Sleep Heart Health Study show prevalences of mild (32%) and moderate-to-severe (19%) OSA in the 60–69-year age group [40]. Based on these data, 51% of people in the 60–69-year age group had an AHI above 5 events per hour, the upper normal value based on current criteria. In comparison, the studies reported an AHI > 5 events per hour in 88% and 59% of the included IPF patients, respectively [9, 29].

These percentages are higher than those seen in this age group in the SHHS. The main difference between the studies in IPF patients is the fact that the majority of patients (68%) had moderate-to-severe OSA (AHI >15 events per hour) [9], compared to (44%) mild OSA (AHI 5–15 events per hour) [29]. These differences may be related to the fact that [29] included only treatment-naïve patients while [9] included patients treated with corticosteroids, which may increase OSA as a result of fat deposition in the neck area. In addition, the body mass index (BMI) of patients in the study [29] was significantly lower than the BMI in the study by [9].

The role of underlying OSA in the general health status of IPF patients is probably more important than has been recognized. There are a few published studies reporting that some features related to OSA, such as increased gastro-esophageal reflux, exaggerated intrathoracic mechanical strains or intermittent hypoxia with oxidative stress, could favor the development of IPF or impact the progression of the disease [18, 32, 41]. OSA is also linked to cardiovascular and cerebrovascular morbidity and mortality [42, 43].

The recent IPF guidelines include OSA among the IPF-associated comorbidities [35]. Up to now only a few studies in IPF patients with CPAP treatment have been available [44].

The first study included 12 IPF patients with moderate-to-severe OSA started on CPAP therapy [33]. Effective CPAP treatment in IPF patients with OSA resulted in a significant improvement in daily living activities based on the Functional Outcome of Sleep Questionnaire (FOSQ), a specific follow-up instrument that assesses the daily effects of poor sleep caused by sleep disorders. A statistically significant improvement was observed in the FOSQ at 1, 3 and 6 months after CPAP initiation. Another study in a cohort of 31 treatment-naïve, newly diagnosed, consecutive IPF patients reported that intermittent sleep oxygen desaturation significantly exceeds that of maximal exercise and is associated with survival in IPF patients [45]. Among the included subjects, 12 (39%) patients had mild and 16 (52%) patients had moderate-to-severe OSA. The main limitation of this study was that only four patients were treated with CPAP.

In a multicenter study CPAP therapy was initiated in 92 treatment-naïve, newly diagnosed, consecutive IPF patients with moderate-to-severe OSA [28]. Patients were divided into a poor and a good CPAP compliance group. All subjects completed multiple quality-of-life and sleep instruments (FOSQ, Pittsburgh Sleep Quality Index, Epworth Sleepiness Scale, Fatigue Severity Scale, Short Form 36 Health Survey and Beck Depression Inventory) before CPAP initiation and 1 year after the start of CPAP treatment. The good CPAP compliance group showed statistically significant improvement in all used quality-of-life and sleep instruments after 1 year of CPAP therapy. During the 24-monthfollow-up period after CPAP initiation, three patients from the poor CPAP compliance group died, whereas all patients from the good CPAP compliance group remained alive. This is the first study to report that effective CPAP treatment in IPF patients with comorbid moderate-to-severe OSA results in a significant improvement in daily living activities, and quality of sleep and life.

The main complaint in IPF patients with OSA is daytime fatigue that is difficult to assess [29, 37]. The majority of the respiratory events are hypopnoeas and the accurate recognition of these needs special equipment and follows new terminology [9, 24, 29, 30].

INFLAMMATORY ROLE OF SLEEP-DISORDERED BREATHING

Episodic intermittent hypoxemia in sleep-disordered breathing stimulates occurrence of significant oxidative stress, systemic vascular endothelial damage, and inflammation [46, 47].

This results in the generation of highly reactive superoxide radicals, which facilitates reperfusion-mediated endothelial injury. Free oxygen radicals released from polymorphonuclear leukocytes during hypoxemic episodes further propagate this vascular oxidative stress. Occurrence of episodic hypoxemia from nocturnal desaturations also activates carotid chemoreceptors, thereby triggering arteriolar vasoconstriction and systemic catecholamine secretion [48].

Serum levels of tumor necrosis factor-α, interleukin-6, and C-reactive protein (CRP) may also be elevated in response to sleep deprivation and hypoxia, both of which occur in OSA and in IPF. CRP mediates the inhibition of nitric oxide synthase, thus leading to an increase in the expression of certain cell adhesion molecules thereby modulating the adhesion of leukocytes to endothelial cells. This may be responsible for elevated levels of cell adhesion molecules in individuals with fibrotic lung disease who experience severe OSA [49-58].

References

[1] Margaritopoulos GA, Romagnoli M, Poletti V et al. Recent advances in the pathogenesis and clinical evaluation of pulmonary fibrosis. *Eur Respir Rev* 2012; 21: 48–56.

[2] Schweisfurth H, Kieslich C, Satake N et al. Wie werden interstitielle Lungenerkrankungen in Deutschland diagnostiziert? Ergebnisse des wissenschaftlichen Registers zur Erforschung von interstitiellen Lungenerkrankungen („Fibroseregister") der WATL. Pneumologie 2003; 57: 373-382.

[3] Schweisfurth H. Idiopathische pulmonale Fibrose (IPF). *Atemw-Lungenkrkh 2013*; 39: 484-490.

[4] Schiza S, Mermigkis C, Margaritopoulos GA et al. Idiopathic pulmonary fibrosis and sleep disorders: no longer strangers in the night. *Eur Respir Rev* 2015; 136: 327-339.

[5] McNicholas WT, Verbraecken J, Marin JM. Sleep disorders in COPD: the forgotten dimension. *Eur Respir Rev* 2013; 22: 365–375.

[6] McNicholas WT. Impact of sleep in COPD. *Chest* 2000; 117: Suppl 2, 48S–53S.

[7] Chaouat A, Weitzenblum E, Krieger J et al. Association of chronic obstructive pulmonary disease and sleep apnea syndrome. *Am J Respir Crit Care Med* 1995; 151: 82–86.

[8] Machado MC, Vollmer WM, Togeiro SM et al. CPAP and survival in moderate-to-severe obstructive sleep apnoea syndrome and hypoxaemic COPD. *Eur Respir J* 2010; 35: 132–137.

[9] Lancaster LH, Mason WR, Parnell JA et al. Obstructive sleep apnea is common in idiopathic pulmonary fibrosis. *Chest.* 2009; 136: 772–778.

[10] Aydogdu M, Ciftci B, Firat Guven S et al. Assessment of sleep with polysomnography in patients with interstitial lung disease. *Tuberkuloz ve Toraks*. 2006; 54: 213–221.

[11] Clark M, Cooper B, Singh S et al. A survey of nocturnal hypoxaemia and health related quality of life in patients with cryptogenic fibrosing alveolitis. *Thorax* 2001; 56: 482–486.

[12] Mermigkis C, Chapman J, Golish J et al. Sleep-related breathing disorders in patients with idiopathic pulmonary fibrosis. *Lung* 2007; 185: 173–178.

[13] Sériès F, Cormier Y, Lampron N et al. Increasing the functional residual capacity may reverse obstructive sleepapnea. *Sleep*1988; 11: 349–353.

[14] Heinzer RC, Stanchina ML, Malhotra A et al. Lung volume and continuous positive airway pressurerequirements in obstructive sleep apnea. *Am J Respir Crit Care Med* 2005; 172: 114–117.

[15] Shepherd KL, Holloway RH, Hillman DR, Eastwood PR. The impact of continuous positive airway pressure on the lower esophageal sphincter. *Am J Physiol Gastrointest Liver Physiol* 2007; 292: G1200–G1205.

[16] Ryerson CJ, Berkeley J, Carrieri-Kohlman VL et al. Depression and functional status are strongly associated with dyspnea in interstitial lung disease. *Chest* 2011; 139: 609–616.

[17] Krishnan V, McCormack MC, Mathai SC et al. Sleep quality and health-related quality of life in idiopathic pulmonary fibrosis. *Chest* 2008; 134: 693–698.

[18] Gusbin N, Fry S, Mallart A, Wallaert B. Idiopathic pulmonary fibrosis and sleep disorders. *Rev Pneumol Clin* 2013; 69: 41-45.

[19] Lederer DJ, Jelic S, Bhattacharya J, Basner RC. Is obstructive sleep apnea a cause of idiopathic pulmonary fibrosis? *Arch Pathol Lab Med* 2012; 136: 470.

[20] Reid T, Vennelle M, McKinley M et al. Sleep-disordered breathing and idiopathic pulmonary fibrosis--is there an association? *Sleep Breath* 2015; 19: 719-721.

[21] Duchna H-W. Sleep-related breathing disorders—a second edition of the International Classification of Sleep Disorders (ICSD-2) of the American Academy of Sleep Medicine (AASM). *Pneumologie* 2006; 60: 568–575.

[22] Sateia M J. International classification of sleep disorders-third edition: highlights and modifications. *Chest* 2014; 146: 1387–1394.

[23] American Thoracic Society/European Respiratory Society international multidisciplinary consensus classification of the idiopathic interstitial pneumonias. *Am J Respir Crit Care Med* 2002; 165: 277–304.

[24] American Academy of Sleep Medicine. The AASM Manual for the scoring of sleep and associated events. *Rules, Terminology and Technical Specifications*. Westchester, AASM, 2014.

[25] Rasche K, Orth MJ. Sleep and breathing in idiopathic pulmonary fibrosis. *Physiol Pharmacol* 2009; 60: Suppl 5,13–14.

[26] Perez-Padilla R, West P, Lertzman M, Kryger MH. Breathing during sleep in patients with interstitial lung disease. *Am Rev Respir Dis* 1985; 132: 224–229.

[27] Bye PTP, Issa F, Berthon-Jones M, Sullivan C E. Studies of oxygenation during sleep in patients with interstitial lung disease. *Am Rev Respir Dis* 1984; 129: 27–32.

[28] Mermigkis C, Bouloukaki I, Antoniou K et al. Obstructive sleep apnea should be treated in patients with idiopathic pulmonary fibrosis. *Sleep Breath* 2015; 19: 385–391.

[29] Mermigkis C, Stagaki E, Tryfon S et al. How common is sleep-disordered breathing in patients with idiopathic pulmonary fibrosis? *Sleep Breath* 2010; 14: 387–390.

[30] Pihtili A, Bingol Z, Kiyan E et al. Obstructive sleep apnea is common in patients with interstitial lung disease. *Sleep Breath* 2013; 17:1281–1288.

[31] Lederer DJ, Jelic S, Basner RC et al. Circulating KL-6, a biomarker of lung injury, in obstructive sleep apnoea. *Eur Respir J* 2009; 33:793–796.

[32] Lederer DJ, Jelic S, Bhattacharya J, Basner RC. Is obstructive sleep apnea a cause of idiopathic pulmonary fibrosis? *Arch Pathol Lab Med* 2012; 136: 470.

[33] Mermigkis C, Bouloukaki I, Antoniou KM et al. CPAP therapy in patients with idiopathic pulmonary fibrosis and obstructive sleep apnea: does it offer a better quality of life and sleep? *Sleep Breath* 2013; 17: 1137–1143.

[34] Mulgrew AT, Fox N, Ayas NT, Ryan CF. Diagnosis and initial management of obstructive sleep apnea without polysomnography: a randomized validation study. *Ann Intern Med* 2007; 146: 157–166.

[35] Raghu G, Collard HR, Egan JJ et al. An official ATS/ERS/JRS/ALAT statement: idiopathic pulmonary fibrosis: evidence-based guidelines for diagnosis and management. *Am J Respir Crit Care Med* 2011; 183: 788–824.

[36] Mermigkis C, Bouloukaki I, Schiza SE. Obstructive sleep apnea in patients with interstitial lung diseases: past and future. *Sleep Breath* 2013; 17: 1127–1128.

[37] Agarwal S, Richardson B, Krishnan V et al. Interstitial lung disease and sleep: what is known? *Sleep Med* 2009; 10: 947–951.

[38] Mermigkis C, Stagaki E, Amfilochiou A et al. Sleep quality and associated daytime consequences in patientswith idiopathic pulmonary fibrosis. *Med Princ Pract* 2009; 18: 10–15.

[39] Sériès F, Cormier Y, Lampron N et al.Influence of lung volume in sleep apnea. *Thorax* 1989; 44: 52–57.

[40] Young T, Shahar E, Nieto FJ et al. Sleep Heart Health Study Research Group Predictors of sleep-disordered breathing in community-dwelling adults: the Sleep Heart Health Study. *Arch Intern Med* 2002; 162: 893-900.

[41] Leslie KO. Idiopathic pulmonary fibrosis may be a disease of recurrent, tractional injury to the periphery of theaging lung: a unifying hypothesis regarding etiology and pathogenesis. *Arch Pathol Lab Med* 2012; 136: 591–600.

[42] Peppard PE, Young T, Palta M et al. Prospective study of the association between sleep-disordered breathing andhypertension. *N Engl J Med* 2000; 342: 1378–1384.

[43] Shahar E, Whitney CW, Redline S et al. Sleep-disordered breathing and cardiovascular disease: cross-sectionalresults of the Sleep Heart Health Study. *Am J Respir Crit Care Med* 2001; 163: 19–34.

[44] Mermigkis C, Mermigkis D, Varouchakis G et al. CPAP treatment in patients with idiopathic pulmonary fibrosisand obstructive sleep apnea—therapeutic difficulties and dilemmas. *Sleep Breath* 2012; 16: 1–3.

[45] Kolilekas L, Manali E, Vlami KA et al. Sleep oxygen desaturation predicts survival in idiopathic pulmonaryfibrosis. *J Clin Sleep Med* 2013; 9: 593–601.

[46] Lévy P, Pépin JL, Arnaud C et al. Intermittent hypoxia and sleep-disordered breathing: current concepts and perspectives. *Euro Respir J* 2008; 32: 1082–1095.

[47] Neubauer JA. Invited review: physiological and pathophysiological responses to intermittent hypoxia. *J Appl Physiol* 2001; 90: 1593–1599.

[48] Adegunsoye A, Balachandran J. Inflammatory response mechanisms exacerbating hypoxemia in coexistent pulmonary fibrosis and sleep

apnea. *Mediators Inflamm.* 2015;2015:510105. doi: 10.1155/2015/510105. Epub 2015 Apr 5.

[49] Kuniyoshi FH, Garcia-Touchard A, Gami AS et al. Day-night variation of acute myocardial infarction in obstructive sleep apnea. *J Am Coll Cardiol* 2008; 52: 343–346.

[50] Parish JM, Somers VK. Obstructive sleep apnea and cardiovascular disease. *Mayo Clinic Proc* 2004; 79: 1036–1046.

[51] Kasasbeh E, Chi DS, Krishnaswamy G. Inflammatory aspects of sleep apnea and their cardiovascular consequences. *South Med J* 2006; 99: 58–67.

[52] Hartmann G, Tschöp M, Fischer R et al. High altitude increases circulating interleukin-6, interleukin-1 receptor antagonist and C-reactive protein. *Cytokine* 2000; 12: 246–252.

[53] Vgontzas AN, Papanicolaou DA, Bixler EO et al. Circadian interleukin-6 secretion and quantity and depth of sleep. *J Clin Endocrinol Meta* 1999; 84: 2603–2607.

[54] Vgontzas AN, Papanicolaou DA, Bixler EO et al. Elevation of plasma cytokines in disorders of excessive daytime sleepiness: role of sleep disturbance and obesity. *J Clin Endocrinol Metab* 1997; 82: 1313–1316.

[55] Shamsuzzaman ASM, Winnicki M, Lanfranchi P et al. Elevated C-reactive protein in patients with obstructive sleep apnea. *Circulation* 2002; 105: 2462–2464.

[56] Venugopal SK, Devaraj S, Yuhanna I et al. Demonstration that C-reactive protein decreases eNOS expression and bioactivity in human aortic endothelial cells. *Circulation* 2002; 106: 1439–1441.

[57] Woollard KJ, Phillips DC, Griffiths HR. Direct modulatory effect of C-reactive protein on primary human monocyte adhesion to human endothelial cells. *Clin Exp Immunol* 2002; 130: 256–262.

[58] Lee RN, Kelly E, Nolan G et al. Disordered breathing during sleep and exercise in idiopathic pulmonary fibrosis. *QJM* 2016; 109: 142.

[59] Andreas S. *Obstructive sleep apnoea: clinical aspects. ERS Handbook Respiratory Sleep Medicine,* ed. Simonds AK, de Backer W, 2012, 32-34.

In: Cystic and Idiopathic Pulmonary Fibrosis ISBN: 978-1-63485-508-2
Editor: Lorenzo Robertson

Chapter 7

N-Acetylcysteine Therapy in Idiopathic Pulmonary Fibrosis

E. Rindone[1], L. Rosset[2,*] and C. Carnuccio[3]

[1]Division of respiratory disease,
Department of Clinical Biological Sciences,
Faculty of Medicine and Surgery, San Luigi Gonzaga,
University of Turin, Turin, Italy
[2]Faculty of Medicine and Surgery, San Luigi Gonzaga,
University of Turin, Turin, Italy
[3]Casa di cura Villa Serena, Piossasco, Turin, Italy

Abstract

Idiopathic pulmonary fibrosis (IPF) is a progressive lung disease determined by dysfunction of epithelial cells. Basically normal parenchyma is subverted into fibrotic tissue useless for gas exchange.

Genetic factors, aging and the exposure to exogenous agents are involved in the beginning of the disorder process. The genetic determination gained importance when plenty of evidences have been highlighted like familial clustering, combination with rare genetic disorders, and variability of IPF onset on individuals with same agents exposures where highlighted. MUC5 B variants are associated with the disorder, while TOLLIP and SPPL2C variants are related to IPF

[*] Corresponding Author address Email: lorenzo_rosset@yahoo.it.

susceptibility and mortality. At the moment, the determination of genetic variants cannot be a routine exam and, at the same time would not be useful in therapy or in prognosis since its role is limited to IPF predisposition.

Predisposition is only the first of the three IPF pathogenesis stages.

The second stage sees the onset of profibrotic processes: the consequences of excessive TGF β activation, Endoplasmic Reticulum stress and growth factors secretion are the epithelial to mesenchymal transition (EMT) and fibrocyte recruitment. The last stage is the progression with pathologic fibroblast differentiation and matrix remodeling ending in epigenetic changes that can feed itself the disease development activating persistently mesenchymal cells and simulating fibrosis progression.

The differentiation stage is useful to determine molecular pathways and address IPF therapies towards specific targets.

Latest studies demonstrated the relationship between N-acetylcysteine (NAC) and EMT, MUC5 ac, MUC5B and TOLLIP. The use of acetylcysteine seems to be favourable in patient's therapy, at least in some genetic cluster. In the light of these latest findings NAC should be reconsidered in IPF therapy.

Keywords: pulmonary, fibrosis, IPF, genetic, pathogenesis, treatment, pirfenidone, nintedanib, NAC, acetylcysteine

INTRODUCTION

Idiopathic pulmonary fibrosis (IPF) is a progressive fibrosing interstitial pneumonia of unidentified cause [1]. It is a lung disease determined by dysfunction of epithelial cells. Basically normal parenchyma is subverted into fibrotic tissue useless for gas exchange causing progressive worsening of dyspnea associated with a poor prognosis [2].

EPIDEMIOLOGY

Idiopathic pulmonary Fibrosis is one of the most common forms of interstitial lung disease (prevalence of 50 per 100,000). The prevalence of IPF rises dramatically with age; it is virtually absent in patients under 50 years of age but is present in an estimated 0.2% of those older than 75.

Idiopathic pulmonary Fibrosis incidence is rising as shown by statistical assessments. In UK 5000 new cases are diagnosed each year and the disease claims the same number of people [3]. In USA the incidence in people aged 65 years and older passed from 93.7/100000/year (2001) to 494.5/100000/year (2011) also the prevalence is substantially higher than previously reported [4].

Mortality has increased in USA and UK, but the major role in this increment could be played by the improvement in IPF diagnosis [5].

Survival and prognosis are worsened by age and comorbidities.

If we look at patients under the age of 65 the median survival is 6.8 years. This data decreases from 4.5 to 1.6 years, respectively in people aged 65–69 years and ≥85 years [3].

Pulmonary hypertension and emphysema, gastro-oesophageal reflux disease and lung cancer are involved into a significant reduction of the survival [5].

GENETIC

Genetic factors, aging and the exposure to exogenous agents are involved in the beginning of the disorder process. The genetic determination gained importance since a lot of evidences have been highlighted like familial clustering, the combination with rare genetic disorders, and variability of IPF onset on individuals with same agents exposures.

MUC5 B is the most important mucine expressed in human airway secretions mainly in bronchus glands and also in submaxillary glands, endocervix, gallbladder, and pancreas [6]. MUC5 B genetic variants and a common single nucleotide polymorphism (SNP) have been associated with interstitial pneumonia and IPF. A linkage between idiopathic interstitial pneumonia and a 3.4-Mb region of chromosome 11p15 was described by Seibold et al. The minor allele (T) of SNP rs35705950, located 3 kb upstream of the MUC5B transcription start site, has been found in 34% subjects with familial interstitial pneumonia, in 38% subjects with IPF, and in 9% controls. MUC5B expression in subjects with IPF was 14.1 times compared to those who did not [7].

Short telomeres are common findings in IPF but also TERT and TERC mutations are proven to be related to sporadic and familial cases of IPF [8].

TOLLIP (Toll Interacting Protein) carries out its ubiquitin-binding protein function regulating immune responses interacting with signaling cascade mediated by Toll-like receptor, transforming growth factor β (TGF-β) and IL-1 [9].

Completed studies apparently had several limitations, TOLLIP variants seem to be associated with IPF susceptibility and the rs5743890 variant is also associated with increased mortality. Furthermore the relation between the reduced expression of the gene and IPF is demonstrated [10].

The question is how can we use these genetics informations?

Today there is no recommendation for any kind of genetic test either in patients diagnosed with IPF or in unaffected family members. The reasons to be considered are: the variable penetrance of dominant mutations, if an early detection of IPF does change the disease course or the patient management and the average cost of genetic tests [11].

PATHOGENESIS

The IPF pathogenesis can be divided into a series of subsequent events grouped in three stages: predisposition, initiation and progression.

The predisposition stage involves: genetic factors, exogenous exposure to environment and aging.

Genetic factors, as seen before, include mutations or variations, for example Single Nucleotide Polymorphism, that predispose individuals to develop the lung disease.

Aging is involved since the chronic epithelial cell turnover leads to shortened telomeres during the life time. All these factors must be kept in mind when the causes of epithelial cell dysfunction are being considered.

At this point we need to remark the fact that not all people who reach this stage will advance to the following stage, but, for sure, the disease progression depends on duration and degree of agents exposure.

The initiation stage includes profibrotic processes like fibrocyte recruitment, and fibroblast differentiation.

Excessive TGF beta activation (a mediator that stimulates fibroblast proliferation and collagen production, and inhibits fibroblast apoptosis) leads to epithelial-to-mesenchymal transition (EMT). EMT is also determined by secretion of growth factor, chemokine, or Wnt (secreted glycoproteins that play key roles in lung development, cancer, and fibrogenesis). The activation of Unfolded Protein Response (UPR), when engaged, accelerates the process Endoplasmic Reticulum stress.

The final progression stage includes pathologic fibroblast differentiation, matrix deposition and remodeling; increased matrix stiffness, and profibrotic epigenetic changes within fibroblast and epithelial cells. These molecular processes lead to fibrosis. The lungs remodeling and scar is determined by pathologic mesenchymal cells release of abnormal types and quantities of matrix proteins.

The resultant remodeled matrix or pathologic fibroblasts could set up persistent mesenchymal cell activation and progressive fibrosis [12].

A high prevalence of abnormal acid gastroesophageal reflux (GER) has been observed in patients with IPF and is considered a risk factor for its development [13].

What about the future?

The future seems to point towards improved knowledge of pathways molecular actions: the relationship between lung profibrotic molecular changes and MUC5B, TERT or TERT mutations; the discovery of other mutations involved in lung fibrosis; the identification of environmental factors and their relationship with IPF pathogenesis, clarify how short telomeres and aging contribute to IPF.

The corner-stone of the problem is understanding whether IPF is a single disorder or if it's a group of diseases that have common phenotypic features with different molecular and/or genetic causes [12].

HISTORY OF N-ACETYLCYSTEINE IN IPF THERAPY

The international guidelines give no strong recommendations for IPF treatment with any drug, but only conditional recommendations with novel agents such as Pirfenidone and Nintedanib.

Pirfenidone is a TGFβ and TNFα regulator that inhibits fibroblast proliferation and collagen deposition. According with ASCEND study, Pirfenidone induces a modest reduction of forced vital capacity (FVC) decline rate compared to placebo. Although an improvement in progression-free survival (PFS) has been demonstrated while there is no difference in overall survival [24].

National Institute for Health and Care Excellence of UK stated that Pirfenidone can be considered an option for treating idiopathic pulmonary fibrosis only if: the person has a FVC between 50% and 80% predicted and the manufacturer provides Pirfenidone with the discount agreed in the patient access scheme.

Instead, if there is evidence of disease progression (FVC decline of 10% or more in 12 months), Pirfenidone should be discontinued. Patients that don't match the guidelines inclusion criteria should continue the treatment until, according with the clinician, they consider it opportune [24, 25].

Nintedanib (BIBF 1120) is an intracellular inhibitor of several tyrosine kinases that targets multiple growth factor receptors like vascular endothelial growth factor, fibroblast growth factor, and platelet-derived growth factor. Different Randomized controlled trials demonstrated the reduction of FVC decline consistent with disease progression slowing, but as Pirfenidone, the overall survival is not improved [26].

Conditional recommendation against Ambrisentan (a selective ER-Aendothelin receptor antagonist), Bosentan or Macitentan (both dual ER-A and ER-B endothelin receptor antagonists) and Sildenafil (a phosphodiesterase-5 inhibitor) are given by statements.

The anti-acid therapy is recommended since it is associated with a slower decline in FVC and a reduced number of acute exacerbations in patients with idiopathic pulmonary fibrosis [1, 13].

There is a strong recommendation against the use of warfarin, imatinib, combination therapy of N-acetylcysteine, azathioprine and prednisone [1].

The use of N-Acetylcysteine is not suggested against what older statements did: ATS/ERS 2011 consensus guidance suggested NAC (alone or in triple therapy) use in a minority of patients and the 2013 NICE guideline suggested that NAC could be used alone after discussion of the treatment risks [1, 27, 28].

Nacetylcysteine is a mucolytic agent that acts both as precursor and reduced antioxidant glutathione (GSH) which could be reduced in the lungs of IPF patients. It is a thiol containing compound which can act as a reduced or precursor glutathione. NAC interferes with different cellular processes like apoptosis, cytokine production and cellular growth [29-32]. GSH carries out its work protecting biological structures and functions [33]. The NAC actions have been proved in laboratory tests and also in vivo.

In 1990 a relationship between IPF and a GSH poor environment for excessive fibroblast proliferation was demonstrated in vitro in bronchoalveolar lavage fluid (BAL) or calf serum (CS) cells [34].

A 1995 study on the glutathione deficiency in lung epithelial lining fluid (ELF) discussed the effects of intravenous NAC in IPF. The Glutathione levels were significantly increased in bronchoalveolar lavage fluid (BALF) and ELF. The study showed that IPF patients can safely improve lung glutathione levels with the help of antioxidant protection [35].

TGF-beta involved in IPF remodeling or fibrotic processes can be affected by NAC in human fetal lung fibroblasts (HFL-1). NAC abolishes gel contraction in vitro and regulates the production of fibronectin and VEGF as important mediators of tissue repair and remodeling [36].

NAC inhibits EMT TGF-beta1 induced and the switch into fibroblast-like morphology in rat epithelial cell line (RLE-6TN) and in primary rat alveolar epithelial cells (AEC) vitro [36].

In IPF or sarcoidosis bronchoalveolar lavage (BAL) cells NAC has got dose-dependent inhibitory effect on the expression of interleukin-8 (IL-8), matrix metalloproteinase-9 (MMP-9) and intercellular cell adhesion molecule-1 (ICAM-1) [37].

N-acetylcysteine inhibits the alveolar macrophages production of TNF-alpha, sTNFR, and TGF-beta1 and the pro-fibrotic and pro-inflammatory actions in IPF affected patient's in vitro culture [38].

NAC can regulate the lysyl oxidase activity alleviating the IPF induced in rats [39].

The p63 total suppression in lung tissues of IPF patients at an early phase was demonstrated using NAC while dexamethasone or pirfenidone showed no effects [40].

The efficacy of NAC mono therapy was evaluated with a multicenter, randomized and controlled clinical trial among patients with early stage IPF. Seventy six patients were randomly assigned to one of two groups: the NAC treatment group and the no therapy group (control). No significant results in the FVC change were shown but a post hoc exploratory analysis associated NAC therapy with FVC stability among patients with initial FVC<95% or initial diffusing capacity of carbon monoxide <55% [41, 42].

Sakamoto's described the difference between two groups: one treated with Pirfenidone and NAC and the other without NAC. After six months the median change in FVC was -290 mL in the non NAC group and 0 mL in the NAC group and the median survival period was 196 ± 57 days in the non NAC group and 557 ± 66 days in the NAC group ($p = 0.03$) [43].

IFIGENIA study compared the regimen consisting of azathioprine, prednisone, and acetylcysteine or without NAC in the IPF therapy. FVC and carbon monoxide diffusing capacity were better preserved using NAC [44]. The PANTHER study investigated the effects of NAC in IPF treatment compared to the three drug therapy. PANTHER was unsafe and so interrupted but an arm of the study continued with NAC monotherapy vs. placebo. Recent study concluded that acetylcysteine did not preserve IPF patients' FVC and it would result in mild-to-moderate impairment in pulmonary function [45].

The effects of combination therapy with inhaled NAC and pirfenidone in advanced IPF has been compared to pirfenidone monotherapy in terms of effectiveness and progression free survival. The combined treatment with pirfenidone and NAC had better outcomes [46].

Genetic and NAC Therapy

NAC regulates MUC5ac and epithelial EMT, phenomena that have not been demonstrated in either pirfenidone or nintedanib treatments [47-49]

Latest studies demonstrated that NAC reduces endpoint risk in genetically predisposed individuals carrying an rs3750920 (TOLLIP) TT genotype. This genotype can be found in 25% of IPF patients, this means that a significant minority could benefit of NAC therapy [50].

On the other side, potential noxiousness in patients with rs3750920 (TOLLIP) CC genotype while no interaction between NAC therapy and rs5743894 (TOLLIP) were observed.

Potential interaction between NAC therapy and rs35705950 within MUC5B was also observed. The rs35705950 polymorphism is linked to MUC5B expression improvement therefore to host defense enhancement [7, 51, 52].

Studies on molecular pathways that determine the stage progression are fundamental for the IPF therapy development. This knowledge is useful to take decision on targeting, but still it is unclear if one target could be enough or if we need to hit different molecular pathways together to reach the goal of an effective therapy.

In conclusion, the genetic of individuals with IPF may determine their NAC therapy response. Nevertheless, considering the lack of differences in side effects, the common off-label therapy of NAC-based therapy can be continued [46, 53, 54].

References

[1] Raghu G, Rochwerg B, Zhang Y, Garcia CA, Azuma A, Behr J, Brozek JL, Collard HR, Cunningham W, Homma S, Johkoh T, Martinez FJ, Myers J, ProtzkoSL, Richeldi L, Rind D, Selman M, Theodore A, Wells AU, Hoogsteden H, Schünemann HJ; American Thoracic Society;

European Respiratory society; Japanese Respiratory Society; Latin American Thoracic Association. An Official ATS/ERS/JRS/ALAT Clinical Practice Guideline: Treatment of Idiopathic Pulmonary Fibrosis. An Update of the 2011 Clinical Practice Guideline. *Am J RespirCrit Care Med.* 2015 Jul 15;192(2):e3-19. doi: 10.1164/rccm.201506-1063ST.

[2] Luppi F, Spagnolo P, Cerri S, Richeldi L. The big clinical trials in idiopathic pulmonary fibrosis. *CurrOpinPulm Med.* 2012 Sep;18(5):428-32. doi: 10.1097/MCP.0b013e3283 567ff9.

[3] Navaratnam V, Fleming KM, West J, Smith CJ, Jenkins RG, Fogarty A, Hubbard RB. The rising incidence of idiopathic pulmonary fibrosis in the U.K. *Thorax.* 2011 Jun;66(6):462-7. doi: 10.1136/thx.2010.148031. Epub 2011 Apr 27.

[4] Raghu G, Chen SY, Yeh WS, Maroni B, Li Q, Lee YC, Collard HR. Idiopathic pulmonary fibrosis in US Medicare beneficiaries aged 65 years and older: incidence, prevalence, and survival, 2001-11. *Lancet Respir Med.* 2014 Jul;2(7):566-72. doi: 10.1016/S2213-2600(14)70101-8. Epub 2014 May 27.

[5] Sgalla G, Biffi A, Richeldi L. Idiopathic pulmonary fibrosis: Diagnosis, epidemiology and natural history. *Respirology.* 2015 Nov 23. doi: 10.1111/resp.12683.

[6] Desseyn JL, Aubert JP, van Seuningen I, Porchet N, Laine A Genomic organization of the 3-prime region of the human mucin gene MUC5B. *J. Biol. Chem.* 272: 16873-16883, 1997.

[7] Seibold MA, Wise AL, Speer MC, Steele MP, Brown KK, Loyd JE, Fingerlin TE, Zhang W, Gudmundsson G, Groshong SD, Evans CM, Garantziotis S, and 17 others. A common MUC5B promoter polymorphism and pulmonary fibrosis. *New Eng. J. Med.* 364: 1503-1512, 2011.

[8] Alder JK, Chen JJ, Lancaster L, Danoff S, Su SC, Cogan JD, Vulto I, Xie M, Qi X, Tuder RM, Phillips JA 3rd, Lansdorp PM, Loyd JE, Armanios MY. Short telomeres are a risk factor for idiopathic pulmonary fibrosis. *ProcNatlAcadSci U S A.* 2008 Sep 2;105(35):13051-6. doi: 10.1073/pnas.0804280105. Epub 2008 Aug 27.

[9] Zhang G, Ghosh S. Negative regulation of toll-like receptor-mediated signaling by Tollip. *J Biol Chem.* 2002 Mar 1;277(9):7059-65. Epub 2001 Dec 18.

[10] Noth I, Zhang Y, Ma SF, Flores C, Barber M, Huang Y, Broderick SM, Wade MS, Hysi P, Scuirba J, Richards TJ, Juan-Guardela BM, Vij R,

Han MK, Martinez FJ, Kossen K, Seiwert SD, Christie JD, Nicolae D, Kaminski N, Garcia JG. Genetic variants associated with idiopathic pulmonary fibrosis susceptibility and mortality: a genome-wide association study. *Lancet Respir Med.* 2013 Jun;1(4):309-17. doi: 10.1016/S2213-2600(13)70045-6. Epub 2013 Apr 17.

[11] Raghu G, Collard HR, Egan JJ, Martinez FJ, Behr J, Brown KK, Colby TV, Cordier JF, Flaherty KR, Lasky JA, Lynch DA, Ryu JH, Swigris JJ, Wells AU, Ancochea J, Bouros D, Carvalho C, Costabel U, Ebina M, Hansell DM, Johkoh T, Kim DS, King TE Jr, Kondoh Y, Myers J, Müller NL, Nicholson AG, Richeldi L, Selman M, Dudden RF, Griss BS, Protzko SL, Schünemann HJ; ATS/ERS/JRS/ALAT Committee on Idiopathic Pulmonary Fibrosis. An official ATS/ERS/JRS/ALAT statement: idiopathic pulmonary fibrosis: evidence-based guidelines for diagnosis and management. *Am J RespirCrit Care Med.* 2011 Mar 15;183(6):788-824. doi: 10.1164/rccm.2009-040GL.

[12] Wolters PJ, Collard HR, Jones KD. Pathogenesis of idiopathic pulmonary fibrosis. *Annu Rev Pathol.* 2014;9:157-79. doi: 10.1146/annurev-pathol-012513-104706. Epub 2013 Sep 13.

[13] Lee JS, Collard HR, Anstrom KJ, Martinez FJ, Noth I, Roberts RS, Yow E, Raghu G; IPFnet Investigators. Anti-acid treatment and disease progression in idiopathic pulmonary fibrosis: ananaly-sis of data from three randomised controlled trials. *Lancet Respir Med.* 2013 Jul;1(5):369-76. doi: 10.1016/S2213-2600(13)70105-X. Epub 2013 Jun 14.

[14] Valeyre D. Towards a better diagnosis of idiopathic pulmonary fibrosis. *Eur Respir Rev.* 2011 Jun;20(120):108-13. doi: 10.1183/ 09059180. 00001611.

[15] Devaraj A. Imaging: how to recognise idiopathic pulmonary fibrosis. *Eur Respir Rev.* 2014 Jun;23(132):215-9. doi: 10.1183/09059180. 00001514.

[16] Gotway MB, Freemer MM, King TE Jr. Challenges in pulmonary fibrosis. 1: Use of high resolution CT scanning of the lung for the evaluation of patientswith idiopathic interstitial pneumonias. *Thorax.* 2007 Jun;62(6):546-53.

[17] Raghu G, Lynch D, Godwin JD, Webb R, Colby TV, Leslie KO, Behr J, Brown KK, Egan JJ, Flaherty KR, Martinez FJ, Wells AU, Shao L, Zhou H, Pedersen PS, Sood R, Montgomery AB, O'Riordan TG. Diagnosis of idiopathic pulmonary fibrosis with high-resolution CT in patients with little or no radiologicalevidence of honeycombing: secondary analysis of

a randomised, controlled trial. *Lancet Respir Med.* 2014 Apr;2(4):277-84. doi: 10.1016/S2213-2600(14)70011-6. Epub 2014 Feb 18.

[18] Maher TM. A clinical approach to diffuse parenchymal lung disease. *Immunol Allergy Clin North Am.* 2012 Nov;32(4):453-72. doi: 10.1016/j.iac.2012.08.004. Epub 2012 Sep 26.

[19] Casoni GL, Tomassetti S, Cavazza A, Colby TV, Dubini A, Ryu JH, Carretta E, Tantalocco P, Piciucchi S, Ravaglia C, Gurioli C, Romagnoli M, Gurioli C, Chilosi M, Poletti V. Transbronchial lung cryobiopsy in the diagnosis of fibrotic interstitial lung diseases. *PLoS One.* 2014 Feb 28;9(2):e86716. doi: 10.1371/journal.pone.0086716. eCollection 2014.

[20] Tomassetti S, Cavazza A, Colby TV, Ryu JH, Nanni O, Scarpi E, Tantalocco P, Buccioli M, Dubini A, Piciucchi S, Ravaglia C, Gurioli C, Casoni GL, Gurioli C, Romagnoli M, Poletti V. Transbronchial biopsy is useful in predicting UIP pattern. *Respir Res.* 2012 Oct 29;13:96. doi: 10.1186/1465-9921-13-96.

[21] Poletti V, Casoni GL, Gurioli C, Ryu JH, Tomassetti S. Lung cryobiopsies: a paradigm shift in diagnostic bronchoscopy? *Respirology.* 2014 Jul;19(5):645-54. doi: 10.1111/resp.12309. Epub 2014 May 26.

[22] Flaherty KR, King TE Jr, Raghu G, Lynch JP 3rd, Colby TV, Travis WD, Gross BH, Kazerooni EA, Toews GB, Long Q, Murray S, Lama VN, Gay SE, Martinez FJ. Idiopathic interstitial pneumonia: what is the effect of a multidisciplinary approach to diagnosis? *Am J RespirCrit Care Med.* 2004 Oct 15;170(8):904-10. Epub 2004 Jul 15.

[23] Tomassetti S, Piciucchi S, Tantalocco P, Dubini A, Poletti V. The multidisciplinary approach in the diagnosis of idiopathic pulmonary fibrosis: a patient case-based review. *Eur Respir Rev.* 2015 Mar;24(135):69-77. doi: 10.1183/09059180.00011714.

[24] King TE Jr, Bradford WZ, Castro-Bernardini S, Fagan EA, Glaspole I, Glassberg MK, Gorina E, Hopkins PM, Kardatzke D, Lancaster L, Lederer DJ, Nathan SD, Pereira CA, Sahn SA, Sussman R, Swigris JJ, Noble PW; ASCEND Study Group. A phase 3 trial of pirfenidone in patients with idiopathic pulmonary fibrosis. *N Engl J Med.* 2014 May 29;370(22):2083-92. doi: 10.1056/NEJMoa1402582. Epub 2014 May 18.

[25] Clarck P, Michaels J, Ashcroft D, Bhatt A, Black A, Bradley M, Campbell I, Chakravarthy U, Cole T, Davidson I, Dervan J, Dixon S, et al. Pirfenidone for treating idiopathic pulmonary fibrosis. *Nice guidance* 24 April 2013.

[26] Richeldi L, du Bois RM, Raghu G, Azuma A, Brown KK, Costabel U, Cottin V, Flaherty KR, Hansell DM, Inoue Y, Kim DS, Kolb M, Nicholson AG, Noble PW, Selman M, Taniguchi H, Brun M, Le Maulf F, Girard M, Stowasser S, Schlenker-Herceg R, Disse B, Collard HR; INPULSIS Trial Investigators. Efficacy and safety of nintedanib in idiopathic pulmonary fibrosis. *N Engl J Med.* 2014 May 29; 370(22):2071-82. doi: 10.1056/NEJMoa1402584. Epub 2014 May 18.

[27] American Thoracic Society. An official ATS/ERS/JRS/ALAT statement: idiopathic pulmonary fibrosis: evidence-based guidelines for diagnosis and management. *Am J Respir Crit Care Med* 2011;183:788–824. http://dx.doi.org/10.1164/rccm.2009-040GL.

[28] National Institute for Health and Care Excellence. Diagnosis and Management of Suspected Idiopathic Pulmonary Fibrosis. Clinical guideline CG163. London: NICE; 2013.

[29] Meyer A, Buhl R, Magnussen H (1994) The effect of oral N-acetylcysteine on lung glutathione levels in idiopathic pulmonary fibrosis. *Eur Respir J* 7: 431-436.

[30] Felton VM, Borok Z, Willis BC (2009) N-acetylcysteine inhibits alveolar epithelial-mesenchymal transition. *Am J Physiol Lung Cell Mol Physiol.* 297: L805-812.

[31] Gillissen A (2011) Anti-inflammatory efficacy of N-acetylcysteine and therapeutic usefulness. *Pneumologie* 65: 549-557.

[32] Adamali HI, Maher TM (2012) Current and novel drug therapies for idiopathic pulmonary fibrosis. *Drug Des Devel Ther* 6: 261-272.

[33] Ruffmann R, Wendel A (1991) GSH rescue by N-acetylcysteine. Klin Wochenschr 69: 857-862. Cantin AM1, Larivée P, Bégin RO (1990) Extracellular glutathione suppresses human lung fibroblast proliferation. *Am J Respir Cell Mol Biol* 3: 79-85.

[34] Cantin AM, Larivée P, Bégin RO (1990) Extracellular glutathione suppresses human lung fibroblast proliferation. *Am J Respir Cell Mol Biol* 3: 79-85.

[35] Meyer A, Buhl R, Kampf S, Magnussen H (1995) Intravenous Nacetylcysteine and lung glutathione of patients with pulmonary fibrosis and normals. *Am J Respir Crit Care Med* 152: 1055-1060.

[36] Sugiura H, Ichikawa T, Liu X, Kobayashi T, Wang XQ, et al. (2009) Nacetyl-L-cysteine inhibits TGF-beta1-induced profibrotic responses in fibroblasts. *Pulm Pharmacol Ther* 22: 487-491.

[37] Radomska-LeÅ›niewska DM, SkopiÅ„ska-RÃ³zewska E, Jankowska Steifer E, Sobiecka M, Sadowska AM, et al. (2010) N-acetylcysteine

inhibits IL-8 and MMP-9 release and ICAM-1 expression by bronchoalveolar cells from interstitial lung disease patients. *Pharmacol Rep* 62: 131-138.

[38] Cu A, Ye Q, Sarria R, Nakamura S, Guzman J, et al. (2009) Nacetylcysteine inhibits TNF-alpha, sTNFR, and TGF-beta1 release by alveolar macrophages in idiopathic pulmonary fibrosis in vitro. Sarcoidosis *Vasc Diffuse Lung Dis* 26: 147-154.

[39] Li S, Yang X, Li W, Li J, Su X, et al. (2012) N-acetylcysteine downregulation of lysyl oxidase activity alleviating bleomycin-induced pulmonary fibrosis in rats. *Respiration* 84: 509-517.

[40] Murata K, Ota S, Niki T, Goto A, Li CP, et al. (2007) p63 - Key molecule in the early phase of epithelial abnormality in idiopathic pulmonary fibrosis. *Exp Mol Pathol* 83: 367-376.

[41] Behr J, Richeldi L (2013) Recommendations on treatment for IPF. *Respir Res;* 14: S6.

[42] Homma S, Azuma A, Taniguchi H, Ogura T, Mochiduki Y, et al. (2012). Efficacy of inhaled N-acetylcysteine monotherapy in patients with early stage idiopathic pulmonary fibrosis. *Respirology* 17: 467-477.

[43] Sakamoto S, Itoh T, Muramatsu Y, Satoh K, Ishida F, et al. (2013). Efficacy of pirfenidone in patients with advanced-stage idiopathic pulmonary fibrosis. *Intern Med* 52: 2495-2501.

[44] Demedts M1, Behr J, Buhl R, Costabel U, Dekhuijzen R, et al. (2005). High-dose acetylcysteine in idiopathic pulmonary fibrosis. *N Engl J Med* 353: 2229-2242.

[45] Idiopathic Pulmonary Fibrosis Clinical Research Network, Martinez FJ, de Andrade JA, Anstrom KJ, King TE Jr, et al. (2014) Randomized trial of acetylcysteine in idiopathic pulmonary fibrosis. *N Engl J Med* 370: 2093-2101.

[46] Sakamoto S, Muramatsu Y, Satoh K, Ishida F, Kikuchi N, Sano G, Sugino K, Isobe K, Takai Y, Homma S. (2015) Effectiveness of combined therapy with pirfenidone and inhaled N-acetylcysteine for advanced idiopathicpulmonary fibrosis: a case-control study. *Respirology.* Apr;20(3):445-52. doi: 10.1111/resp.12477. Epub 2015 Feb 2.

[47] Mata M, Ruı ´z A, Cerda ´ M, Martinez-Losa M, Cortijo J, Santangelo F, et al. (2003) Oral N-acetylcysteine reduces bleomycininduced lung damage and mucin Muc5ac expression in rats. EurRespir J.; 22: 9005.

[48] Felton VM, Borok Z, Willis BC. (2009) N-acetylcysteine inhibits alveolar epithelial-mesenchymal transition. *Am J Physiol Lung Cell Mol Physiol*; 297: L80512.

[49] Myllärniemi M, Kaarteenaho R. (2015) Pharmacological treatment of idiopathic pulmonary fibrosis - preclinical and clinical studies of pirfenidone, nintedanib, and N-acetylcysteine. *Eur Clin Respir J.* 2015 Feb 10;2. doi: 10.3402/ecrj.v2.26385.

[50] Oldham JM, Ma SF, Martinez FJ, Anstrom KJ, Raghu G, Schwartz DA, Valenzi E, Witt L, Lee C, Vij R, Huang Y, Strek ME, Noth I; IPFnet Investigators. (2015). TOLLIP, MUC5B, and the Response to N-Acetylcysteine among Individuals with Idiopathic Pulmonary Fibrosis. *Am J Respir Crit Care Med.* Dec 15;192(12):1475-82. doi: 10.1164/rccm.201505-1010OC.

[51] Molyneaux PL, Cox MJ, Willis-Owen SA, Mallia P, Russell KE, Russell AM, Murphy E, Johnston SL, Schwartz DA, Wells AU, et al. (2014) The role of bacteria in the pathogenesis and progression of idiopathic pulmonary fibrosis. Am J Respir Crit Care Med;190:906–913.

[52] Roy MG, Livraghi-Butrico A, Fletcher AA, McElwee MM, Evans SE, Boerner RM, Alexander SN, Bellinghausen LK, Song AS, Petrova YM, et al. (2014) Muc5b is required for airway defence. *Nature*; 505: 412–416.

[53] Rindone E, Rosset L. The Point on N-acetylcysteine in Idiopathic Pulmonary Fibrosis Treatment. *J Palliat Care Med* 2014 4:193. doi: 10.4172/2165-7386.1000193 2014.

[54] Behr J, Kreuter M, Hoeper MM, Wirtz H, Klotsche J, Koschel D, Andreas S, Claussen M, Groh ´ e C, Wilkens H, et al. (2015) Management of patients with idiopathic pulmonary fibrosis in clinical practice: the INSIGHTS-IPF registry. *Eur Respir J*;46:186–196.

INDEX

B

C

D

E

F

G

H

I

N

O

P

Q

R

U

V

W